Anti Inflammatory Diet Cookbook

The 3 Week Action Plan – 120+ easy to follow recipes and proven meal plan to beat inflammation and for lasting body health

John Carter

Text Copyright © John Carter

evaluated by the U.S Food & Drug Administration, and it is not intended to diagnose, treat, cure or prevent any disease. Full medical clearance from a licensed physician should be obtained before beginning or modifying any diet, exercise or lifestyle program, and physician should be informed of all nutritional changes. The author claims no responsibility to any person or entity for any liability, loss, damage or death caused or alleged to be caused directly or indirectly as a result of the use, application or interpretation of the information presented herein.

Table of Content

5

INTRODUCTION

Toxins are integral part of our environment; they are present in air, water and simply everywhere. No matter how precautionary you are, these toxins, allergens and environmental pollutants find their way into your body. Inflammation is an auto-immune response of our body to fight-off these toxins and pollutants.

Acute and chronic are two major types of inflammation that can be triggers by hundreds of different factors. Our health can be severely affected due to both chronic and acute inflammation. Every year, millions of people fall victim to arthritis; it is a major disease caused by body inflammation. Psoriasis, ulcerative colitis, lupus, hepatitis, sinusitis, arthritis, join pain, sore throat, peptic ulcer, asthma, and flue are other major health complications triggered by body inflammation.

We can't control these allergens, toxins and pollutants, but we can control our diet. Whole foods have amazing healing power to nourish our body from within. Inflammation fighting foods are nutritionally balanced, and play a vital role to keep harmful effects of inflammation at bay.

Rising popularity of anti-inflammatory diet is self-explanatory given its health transforming abilities. The diet has been the center of attention for hundreds of health institutions and dietary clinics across the world. The anti-inflammatory nutrition can be an overwhelming area for many of you. There is nothing complex about managing body inflammation, you can easily make dietary changes without complex nutritional calculations.

Anti-inflammatory diet emphasizes on making healthy changes in your present diet. It includes healthy fruits, green vegetables, healthy cooking oils, and health fats to keep inflammation at bay. Following sections of the book provide a glance about the health benefits of the diet, best foods to eat, foods to avoid, and tips to make healthy lifestyle changes.

Explore nutrition-dense, inflammation fighting recipes in this exclusive anti-inflammatory cookbook. The recipes are packed with wholesome ingredients, and are easy to prepare at home. This book includes a 3-week diet plan along with an action plan; it greatly helps to follow the diet for a long time.

Get ready to learn making these wholesome meals and take control over inflammation. They are your secret to live a fulfilling, happy life.

A GLANCE AT AN ANTI-INFLAMMATORY DIET

WHAT IS BODY INFLAMMATION?

Inflammation is not necessarily a bad thing. As mentioned earlier, it is our body's natural reaction to external stimuli. It can be triggered by many forms of stimuli including bacteria, viruses, fungi, chemicals, allergens, environmental toxins, certain medicinal drugs, and injury to any body part. Inflammation can also be triggered by many lifestyle factors including obesity, smoking, excessive alcohol consumption, nutrient-less diet, and chronic stress.

Our immune system works in co-ordination with many other systems within our body. They form an interconnected network to complete hundreds of routine body functions. Immune system protects our body from any form of external attack; when it senses any possibility of an attach, it produces histamines and other substances to counteract it. Such histamine production often leads to pain, redness, and swelling.

Body inflammation is a strictly regulated process and it must remain under control. When it goes out of control, it starts putting our health at risk. It can be harmful and damaging to healthy tissues. That is why, inflammation should be temporary, and not permanent. Common signs of inflammation include swelling, redness, and or warming sensations around various body parts and joints. Inflammation also includes possible signs of numbness and pain.

Acute inflammation is our body's natural response to repair and heal damaged tissues. It aims at quickly cleansing our body of external stimuli. Acute inflammation is a temporary phenomenon. Chronic inflammation is not temporary; its duration varies from weeks to months. It not controlled, it can create an enormous amount of immune cells, which can lead to the development of many serious illnesses.

WHY YOU MUST CONTROL IT?

If not controlled or prevented, both acute and chronic inflammation can lead to critical health disorders to totally disrupt your lifestyle. Major critical complications include

- Carpal tunnel syndrome

- Alzheimer's disease

- Psoriasis

- Crohn's disease

- Heart attacks,

- Certain types of cancer

- Strokes

- Colitis

- Lupus

- Anemia

- Asthma

- Diabetes

- Rheumatoid arthritis

- Depression (in severe cases)

SMART TIPS FOR AN INFLAMMATION FREE LIFESTYLE

Apart from a healthy diet, you can make small, effective changes in your lifestyle to give a strong punch to inflammatory triggers. These small changes help your body to develop strong resistance against external attacks.

>> PROPER HYDRATION

The importance of water in our life is well-known. It allows us to get rid of waste products (including toxins and allergens) through kidneys. Water is a key liquid component that lubricates numerous body joints. It greatly helps to maintain an ideal health of body joints. A properly hydrated state of our body prevents the development of many inflammatory conditions. Ensure that you are keeping your body ideally hydrated by drinking plenty of water every day.

Drink at least 6-8 glasses (about 1.5 - 2 liters) of water every day to ensure optimum body hydration. Even a mild to moderate level of dehydration can cause inflammatory response or can worsen inflammation symptoms.

>> THE DIET MANAGEMENT

When you are on a mission to beat inflammation; it calls for adapting a smart dietary approach. The key is to achieve the right balance of nutrients in every day diet.

Antioxidants

Found in wholesome vegetables and fruits; they are helpful in inhibiting cell damage. They protect against inflammation and the development of Rheumatoid Arthritis.

Healthy fats

Healthy fats are essential part of any inflammation preventing diet. Healthy fats, including omega-3 fatty acids, assist to reduce inflammation. They are capable of effectively managing the symptoms of depression.

Minerals

Fresh vegetables, leafy greens, nuts, seeds etc. are high with essential minerals such as zinc, magnesium, potassium, and calcium. Processed foods and commercially packed foods lack essential minerals; they contain high amount of additives and preservatives to trigger inflammatory response. Modern-day farming practices have also contributed in the process of soil demineralization. As a result, plants are receiving less nutrition from soil.

Vitamins

Vitamins are important anti-oxidation supporters. Vitamin C helps to build collagen and repair joints. Vitamin D is known to improve bone health, and fight off inflammatory response caused by environmental allergens. Vitamin E helps to increase the production of essential cartilages in our body. Vitamin D, also referred as the "sunshine vitamin," assists to suppress the auto immune response. Moreover, it helps to control depression symptoms.

>> EXERCISE & SLEEP

Sedentary lifestyle is definitely not a great sign for anyone. If not managed in time, it can send invitations to many health complications. Mild to moderate exercise/jogging is greatly helpful to enhance the effects of anti-inflammatory diet. Even a brief 15-30 minutes of mild exercise/jogging is highly effective. You can also opt for yoga classes.

Give proper rest to your body; sleep is a great nourisher of your holistic health. Make sure that you are taking 7-8 hours of relaxing sleep every night. Hit the sack at reasonable sleeping hours. Your bedtime is also an important factor. Make a habit of switching off all electronics at least one hour before your bedtime.

In order to maintain a hassle-free meal planning, list down all the required ingredients and purchase them in one grocery store visit. Ingredients having larger pantry life can be purchased in higher quantity.

FOODS TO EAT

Anti-inflammatory diet helps to calm down our body's immune response to allergic reactions. It combats the harmful effects triggers by the exposure of toxins, allergens, bacteria, viruses, and fungi. Following are the list of inflammation fighting ingredients.

- Omega-3 fatty acids (healthy fats). They are found in eggs, wild caught fish, and grass-fed or pasture raised meat cuts.

- Nuts and seeds such as sunflower seeds, pumpkin seeds, chia seeds, almonds, walnuts, cashews, pistachio etc.

- Onions, ginger, garlic, bell peppers, pumpkin and leeks.

- Green leafy vegetables such as spinach, kale, broccoli, cauliflower, asparagus, Bok Choy etc.

- Herbs such as rosemary, basil, oregano, parsley etc.

- All types of berries, pineapple, apple, oranges, red grapes etc.

- Whole grains such as brown rice, millets, quinoa, and oats.

- Healthy oils such as coconut oil, extra-virgin olive oil, avocado oil, and sesame oil.

- Lentils, beets, avocado, green tea, coconut, mushrooms, zucchini, and beans.

- Spices such as turmeric, cinnamon, black pepper, cumin etc.

- Non-dairy milks such as almond milk, coconut milk etc.

- Red wine (In moderation).

- Honey, maple syrup, dark chocolate, and cacao powder.

FOODS TO AVOID

Following inflammation triggering foods must be avoided. Eliminate them from every day diet and clear them off your pantry shelves.

- Processes meats: They are loaded with saturated fats (sausage, hot dogs, burgers, steaks etc.)

- Unhealthy fats including lard, margarine, and shortening.

- Sugar added products (except for natural fruits): All canned products with added sugars such as soups, canned fruits, yogurts, bars etc.

- Unsweetened canned fruits, tomatoes, etc. should be consumed in moderation.

- Sugar based commercial drinks, beverages, and fruit juices.

- All processed and packaged foods: They are high with additives, artificial colors, and preservatives.

- Refined carbohydrates including white breads, white pasta, and noodles.

- Foods containing trans fats: Commercially processed foods, fried foods, candies, ice creams, and baked items (cookies, crackers, pastries, cakes, muffins etc.)

- Alcoholic beverages.

3-WEEK DIET PLAN& ACTION PLAN

Making a perfect diet plan is all about consuming breakfast and other meals with as much variety as possible. It keeps your everyday diet exciting with various flavors to enjoy. Following is a sample diet plan for 21 days (3 weeks).

Few action plans to keep in mind.

>> It is not compulsory to stick to the following meal plan. If you crave to eat any particular recipe on a given day, you can replace it. Your diet plan is perfect as long as you are including anti-inflammatory recipes.

>> For lunch, the book includes many salad and soup recipes. Lunch is a light meal and some people like to have a salad or soup. In order to keep it simple, you can choose any soup or salad recipe from the below list. That way, you will have 3 options every day to choose for lunch.

Soup and salad recipes for lunch.

- Fruit Blast Salad

- Avocado Quinoa Salad

- Pomegranate Kale Salad

- Turkey Green Salad

- Chicken Swiss Salad

- Chicken Spinach Salad

- Mushroom Lentil Soup

- Chicken Jalapeno Soup

- Broccoli Potato Soup

- Yogurt Tomato Soup

- Coconut Avocado Soup

- Spinach Mushroom Soup

>> Smoothies are complimentary to have along with morning breakfast. You can choose to have both breakfast and smoothie, or just breakfast.

>> Many people like to have just juice or smoothie as breakfast. Having just smoothie or juice for breakfast is also a perfectly healthy choice.

>> Appetizer and sides are totally optional. Some people like to have some veggies along with their meals. It totally depends on your preference.

>> Snack and desserts are also optional. Having a snack between lunch and dinner is an optional choice.

>> Desserts depend on your cravings. You can choose it to have as per your preference.

Day 1	
Breakfast	Cinnamon Banana Pancakes and/or Mint Summer Smoothie
Appetizer/Sides	Salmon Bites
Lunch	Beef Yogurt Meatballs or your choice of salad or your choice of soup
Snack	Cashew Ginger Dip
Dinner	Pork Chili Stew or Zucchini Jalapeno Pork Meal or Coconut Chili Salmon
Dessert	Quinoa Dessert Bars

Day 2	
Breakfast	Mushroom Spinach Frittata and/or Kale Pistachio Smoothie
Appetizer/Sides	Sesame Bok Choy Side
Lunch	Classic Italian Spiced Chicken or your choice of salad or your choice of soup
Snack	Zucchini Crisps
Dinner	Chicken Veggie Dinner Soup or Avocado Pineapple Pork
Dessert	Lemon Coconut Mousse

Day 3	
Breakfast	Ginger Spiced Oats and/or Fig Yogurt Smoothie
Appetizer/Sides	Baked Beet Sides
Lunch	Lamb Garlic Kebabs With Greens/Rice or your choice of salad or your choice of soup
Snack	Bean Potato Spread
Dinner	Beef Bread-Less Meatloaf or Herbed Mussels Treat
Dessert	Cherry Cobbler
Day 4	
Breakfast	Strawberry Chia Breakfast and/or Carrot Pineapple Juice
Appetizer/Sides	Spinach Stuffed Mushrooms
Lunch	Shrimp Mushroom Squash or your choice of salad or your choice of soup
Snack	Honey Bean Dip
Dinner	Tuna Potato Stew or Nutty Pork Steak
Dessert	Spiced Fruit Blast

Day 5	
Breakfast	Pepper Egg Breakfast and/or Pumpkin Cinnamon Smoothie
Appetizer/Sides	Potato Zucchini Appetizers
Lunch	Brown Rice Chicken Meal or your choice of salad or your choice of soup
Snack	Avocado Prosciutto Snack
Dinner	Brussels Chicken Meal or Black Bean Chili Potato
Dessert	Blackberry Granita

Day 6	
Breakfast	Coconut Crepes and/or Pumpkin Cinnamon Smoothie
Appetizer/Sides	Garlic Cauliflower
Lunch	Brown Rice Chicken Meal/ Salmon Broccoli Bowl or your choice of salad or your choice of soup
Snack	Evening Chicken Bites
Dinner	Orange Peas Chicken or Scrumptious Coconut Shrimps
Dessert	Apple Pear Delight

Day 7	
Breakfast	Apple Oats Granola and/or Avocado Cocoa Smoothie
Appetizer/Sides	Lentil Potato Patties
Lunch	Chickpea Lettuce Wraps or your choice of salad or your choice of soup
Snack	Buckwheat Evening Delight
Dinner	Garlic Basil Pork Chops or Fish Shrimp Soup
Dessert	Pumpkin Pecan Treat

Day 8	
Breakfast	Classic Banana Almond Pancakes and/or Fig Yogurt Smoothie
Appetizer/Sides	Potato Zucchini Appetizers
Lunch	Cinnamon Pork Chops or your choice of salad or your choice of soup
Snack	Evening Chicken Bites
Dinner	Couscous Carrot Chicken or Kale Cod Secret
Dessert	Lemon Coconut Mousse

Day 9	
Breakfast	Quinoa Blueberry Bowl and/or Mint Summer Smoothie
Appetizer/Sides	Spinach Stuffed Mushrooms
Lunch	Turkey Lunch Wraps/Cups or your choice of salad or your choice of soup
Snack	Avocado Prosciutto Snack
Dinner	Berry Chops Dinner or Herbed Tomato Chops
Dessert	Quinoa Dessert Bars

Day 10	
Breakfast	Cheddar Spinach Frittata and/or Kale Pistachio Smoothie
Appetizer/Sides	Baked Beet Sides
Lunch	Spinach Sea Bass Lunch or your choice of salad or your choice of soup
Snack	Zucchini Crisps
Dinner	Artichoke Chicken Stew or Chickpea Raisin Curry
Dessert	Apple Pear Delight

Day 11	
Breakfast	Ginger Spiced Oats and/or Turmeric Cinnamon Hot Milk
Appetizer/Sides	Sesame Bok Choy Side
Lunch	Oregano Lettuce Shrimp/ Mexican Pepper Salmon or your choice of salad or your choice of soup
Snack	Bean Potato Spread
Dinner	Spinach Baked Chicken or Honey Scallops
Dessert	Pumpkin Pecan Treat

Day 12	
Breakfast	Cinnamon Banana Pancakes and/or Kale Pistachio Smoothie
Appetizer/Sides	Garlic Cauliflower
Lunch	Mushroom Rice Bowl or your choice of salad or your choice of soup
Snack	Honey Bean Dip
Dinner	Fish Shrimp Soup or Bean Chicken Chili
Dessert	Blackberry Granita

Day 13	
Breakfast	Mushroom Spinach Frittata and/or Carrot Pineapple Juice
Appetizer/Sides	Salmon Bites
Lunch	Mustard Lamb Lunch or your choice of salad or your choice of soup
Snack	Zucchini Crisps
Dinner	Shrimp Scallops Stew or Cauliflower Lamb Meal or Avocado Pineapple Pork
Dessert	Spiced Fruit Blast

Day 14	
Breakfast	Hemp Chia Porridge and/or Kale Pistachio Smoothie
Appetizer/Sides	Lentil Potato Patties
Lunch	Garlic Cod Meal or your choice of salad or your choice of soup
Snack	Bean Potato Spread
Dinner	Sweet Potato Whole Chicken or Beet Haddock Dinner
Dessert	Cherry Cobbler

Day 15	
Breakfast	Pepper Egg Breakfast and/or Mint Summer Smoothie
Appetizer/Sides	Garlic Tomato Sides
Lunch	Cauliflower Coconut Curry or your choice of salad or your choice of soup
Snack	Cashew Ginger Dip
Dinner	Brussels Chicken Meal OrZucchini Buckwheat Pasta
Dessert	Lemon Coconut Mousse

Day 16	
Breakfast	Strawberry Chia Breakfast and/or Turmeric Cinnamon Hot Milk
Appetizer/Sides	Awesome Asparagus
Lunch	Broccoli Chicken Light Casserole or your choice of salad or your choice of soup
Snack	Buckwheat Evening Delight
Dinner	Sprouts Pork Soup or Grilled Mint Chops or Apple Pork Raisins
Dessert	Quinoa Dessert Bars

Day 17	
Breakfast	Coconut Crepes and/or Fig Yogurt Smoothie
Appetizer/Sides	Garlic Kale Sides
Lunch	Cod Cucumber Delight or your choice of salad or your choice of soup
Snack	Spiced Chickpeas
Dinner	Bean Chicken Chili or Bok Choy Steak Dinner
Dessert	Apple Pear Delight

Day 18	
Breakfast	Apple Oats Granola and/or Avocado Cocoa Smoothie
Appetizer/Sides	Potato Zucchini Appetizers
Lunch	Chickpea Patties or your choice of salad or your choice of soup
Snack	Evening Chicken Bites
Dinner	Herbed Broccoli Chicken or Fennel Baked Cod
Dessert	Pumpkin Pecan Treat

Day 19	
Breakfast	Classic Banana Almond Pancakes and/or Pumpkin Cinnamon Smoothie
Appetizer/Sides	Spinach Stuffed Mushrooms
Lunch	Cinnamon Pork Chops or your choice of salad or your choice of soup
Snack	Avocado Prosciutto Snack
Dinner	Chicken White Bean Soup or Stuffed Pepper Delight
Dessert	Blackberry Granita

Day 20	
Breakfast	Classic Banana Almond Pancakes and/or Cherry Beet Smoothie
Appetizer/Sides	Baked Beet Sides
Lunch	Salmon Greens or your choice of salad or your choice of soup
Snack	Honey Bean Dip
Dinner	Sprouts Pork Chops or Brown Rice Lentils
Dessert	Spiced Fruit Blast

Day 21	
Breakfast	Quinoa Blueberry Bowl and/or Pineapple Lush Red Smoothie
Appetizer/Sides	Sesame Bok Choy Side
Lunch	Chickpea Veggie Lunch or your choice of salad or your choice of soup
Snack	Zucchini Crisps
Dinner	Eggplant Pork Stew or Orange Peas Chicken or Fish Curry Dinner
Dessert	Cherry Cobbler

Breakfast
&
Smoothies

Mushroom Spinach Frittata

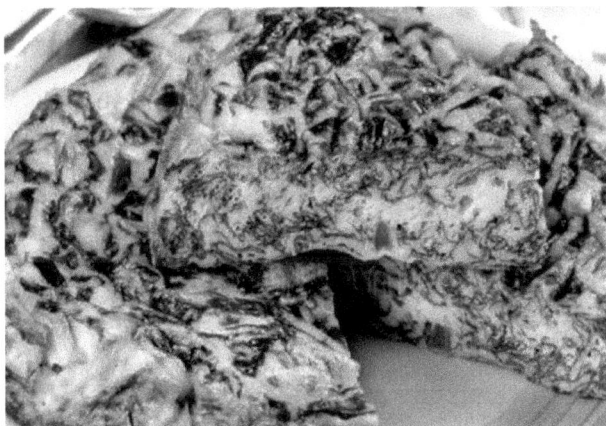

Recipe Time: 25 minutes

Serving Size: 4

Diet Type: Gluten Free, Soy Free, Dairy Free, Nut Free

Ingredients:

- 2 tablespoons avocado or coconut oil
- 8 eggs
- 2 leeks, finely chopped
- ½ teaspoon garlic powder
- ½ teaspoon dried basil
- 1 cup cremini mushrooms, (cut into slices)
- 1 cup baby spinach leaves
- Ground black pepper to taste
- ¾ teaspoon salt

Cooking Instructions:

1. Preheat an oven to 400°F.

2. Take an ovenproof skillet or saucepan (large size). In the skillet or saucepan, heat the oil over medium-high flame.

3. Add the leeks and sauté the leeks, while stirring, for about 5 minutes until turn softened.

4. Take a mixing bowl, whisk the eggs. Add the salt, garlic powder, and basil; combine well.

5. Add the bowl mixture over the leeks; stir-cook for 4-5 minutes.

6. Add the spinach and mushrooms; combine the mixture. Season with black pepper.

7. Transfer the skillet/saucepan to the oven. Bake for 10 minutes, or until the eggs are cooked well.

8. Divide into serving plates and serve warm.

Nutritional Values (Per Serving):

Calories 264, Fat 16g, Carbohydrates 17g, Fiber 3g, Protein 19g

Cinnamon Banana Pancakes

Recipe Time: 15 minutes

Serving Size: 2

Diet Type: Gluten Free, Dairy Free, Soy Free, Nut Free

Ingredients:

- 2 eggs
- 1 egg white
- 1 cup rolled oats
- 1 ripe banana, peeled
- 2 teaspoons ground cinnamon
- 1 teaspoon vanilla extract
- ½ teaspoon salt
- 1 tablespoon coconut oil

Cooking Instructions:

1. In a blender, add the oats and grind to make a coarse flour. Add the egg white, banana, eggs, cinnamon, vanilla, and salt. Blend to make a smooth batter.

2. In a skillet (you can also use a saucepan); heat ½ tablespoon oil over medium stove flame.

3. Add half the batter into the pan to spread evenly. Cook for about 2 minutes until small bubbles form. Flip and cook the other side for about 2 minutes.

4. Repeat the same with remaining batter and serve warm.

Nutritional Values (Per Serving):

Calories 248, Fat 7g, Carbohydrates 31g, Fiber 8g, Protein 12g

Ginger Spiced Oats

Recipe Time: 15-20 minutes

Serving Size: 4

Diet Type: Gluten Free, Dairy Free, Soy Free, Nut Free, Vegan, Vegetarian

Ingredients:

- ¼ teaspoon coriander, ground
- 1 ½ tablespoons cinnamon powder
- ¼ teaspoon cloves, ground
- 1 cup oats, steel cut
- 4 cups water
- ¼ teaspoon allspice, ground
- ¼ teaspoon cardamom, ground
- ¼ teaspoon ginger, grated
- A pinch of nutmeg, ground

Cooking Instructions:

1. In a skillet (you can also use a saucepan); heat the water over medium stove flame.
2. Add the oats and stir the mix.

3. Add the cloves, ginger, allspice, coriander, cinnamon, cardamom and nutmeg, stir, cook for 15 minutes.

4. Add into bowls and serve warm.

Nutritional Values (Per Serving):

Calories 179, Fat 3g, Carbohydrates 13g, Fiber 5g, Protein 6g

Turmeric Cinnamon Hot Milk

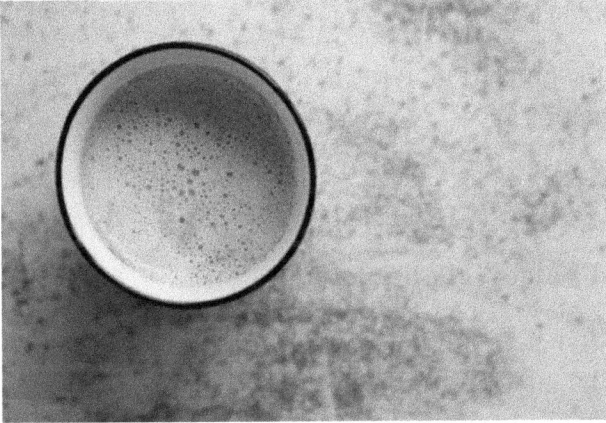

Recipe Time: 5 minutes

Serving Size:2

Diet Type: Gluten Free, Dairy Free, Soy Free, Vegan, Vegetarian

Ingredients:

- ¼ teaspoon ginger, ground
- 1 ½ teaspoon turmeric powder
- 1 ½ cups coconut milk
- 1 ½ cups almond milk
- 1 tablespoon coconut oil
- ¼ teaspoon cinnamon powder

Cooking Instructions:

1. In a skillet (you can also use a saucepan); heat the milks over medium stove flame.

2. Add the ginger, oil, turmeric and cinnamon; stir and cook for 5 minutes.

3. Serve warm.

Nutritional Values (Per Serving):

Calories 168, Fat 3g, Carbohydrates 7g, Fiber 4g, Protein 6g

Cheddar Spinach Frittata

Recipe Time: 35 minutes

Serving Size: 4

Diet Type: Gluten Free, Soy Free

Ingredients:

- ¼ cup coconut milk
- 1 yellow onion, chopped
- 4 ounces white mushrooms, (cut into slices)
- 2 tablespoons olive oil
- 2 cups chopped spinach
- 1 cup cheddar cheese, (shredded or grated)
- 6 eggs
- A pinch of (ground) black pepper and salt

Cooking Instructions:

1. In a skillet (you can also use a saucepan); heat the oil over medium stove flame.
2. Add the onions, stir the mixture and cook while stirring for about 3 minutes until softened.
3. Add the mushrooms, salt and pepper, stir and cook for 2 minutes more.
4. In a bowl (medium size), mix the eggs, cheese, pepper, and salt. Add the mix over the mushrooms.

5. Add the spinach, toss the mixture.

6. Preheat an oven to 360°F.

7. Add the skillet to the oven and bake for 25 minutes. Slice and serve the frittata.

Nutritional Values (Per Serving):

Calories 204, Fat 3g, Carbohydrates 16g, Fiber 6g, Protein 6g

Quinoa Blueberry Bowl

Recipe Time: 5 minutes

Serving Size: 2

Diet Type: Gluten Free, Dairy Free, Soy Free, Vegetarian

Ingredients:

- 2 cups quinoa, cooked
- ¼ cup walnuts, chopped and toasted
- 1 cup cashew or almond milk, warm
- 1 cup blueberries
- 2 teaspoons raw honey
- ½ teaspoon cinnamon powder
- 1 tablespoon chia seeds

Cooking Instructions:

1. In a bowl (medium size), mix the warm milk with the walnuts, honey, blueberries, quinoa, cinnamon and chia seeds.
2. Combine well.
3. Add into serving bowls and serve.

Nutritional Values (Per Serving):

Calories 146, Fat 2g, Carbohydrates 14g, Fiber 5g, Protein 6g

Classic Banana Almond Pancakes

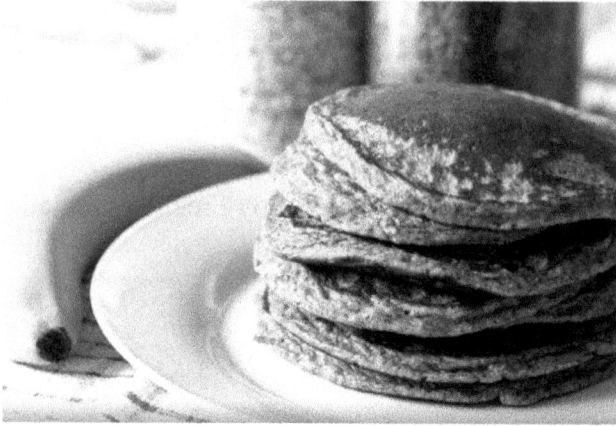

Recipe Time: 10-15 minutes

Serving Size: 4

Diet Type: Gluten Free, Dairy Free, Soy Free

Ingredients:

- 1 teaspoon baking soda
- 3 eggs, beaten
- ½ cup almond flour
- ¼ cup coconut flour
- 2 bananas, peeled and mashed
- 1 teaspoon pure vanilla extract
- 1 tablespoon coconut oil
- Pure maple syrup to taste (optional)

Cooking Instructions:

1. In a bowl (medium size), combine together the flours, and baking soda until well mixed.

2. Make a well in the center and add the bananas, eggs, and vanilla. Combine the mix again.

3. In a skillet (you can also use a saucepan); heat 1/4th oil over medium stove flame.

4. Pour ¼ cup of batter and spread evenly.

5. Cook for about 3 minutes, until bubbles form on the surface. Flip and cook for about 2 minutes more.

   Repeat with the remaining batter. Serve with a drizzle of maple syrup.

Nutritional Values (Per Serving):

Calories 127, Fat 7g, Carbohydrates 9g, Fiber 3g, Protein 5g

Apple Oats Granola

Recipe Time: 45 minutes

Serving Size: 6

Diet Type: Gluten Free, Dairy Free, Soy Free, Nut Free, Vegan, Vegetarian

Ingredients:

- 1 cup sunflower seeds
- 1 cup pumpkin seeds
- 2 cups oats
- 1 cup buckwheat
- 1cup apple puree
- 1 ½ cups dates, pitted and chopped
- 6 tablespoons coconut oil
- 5 tablespoons cocoa powder
- 1 teaspoon ginger, (shredded or grated)

Cooking Instructions:

1. Preheat an oven to 360°F.
2. In a mixing bowl, mix the dates, apple puree, oil, buckwheat, oats, seeds, cocoa powder and ginger.

3. Add over a lined baking sheet, press well to make it of even thickness.

4. Bake for 45 minutes or until cooks well.

5. Slice and serve warm.

Nutritional Values (Per Serving):

Calories 168, Fat 3g, Carbohydrates 12g, Fiber 3g, Protein 7g

Coconut Crepes

Recipe Time: 20-25 minutes

Serving Size: 4

Diet Type: Gluten Free, Dairy Free, Soy Free

Ingredients:

- ½ cup almond milk
- ½ cup water
- 2 eggs
- 1 teaspoon vanilla extract
- 2 tablespoons maple syrup or agave nectar
- 1 cup coconut flour
- 3 tablespoons coconut oil

Cooking Instructions:

1. In a bowl (medium size), mix the eggs. Add the vanilla extract, milk, water and sweetener, and whisk well.
2. Add the flour and 1 tablespoon oil; combine to make a smooth batter.
3. In a skillet (you can also use a saucepan); heat ¼ tablespoon oil over medium stove flame.
4. Pour ¼ cup of batter and spread evenly.

5. Cook until turns light brown. Flip and cook until turns light brown.
   Repeat with the remaining batter.

Nutritional Values (Per Serving):

Calories 132, Fat 3g, Carbohydrates 13g, Fiber 5g, Protein 6g

Strawberry Chia Breakfast

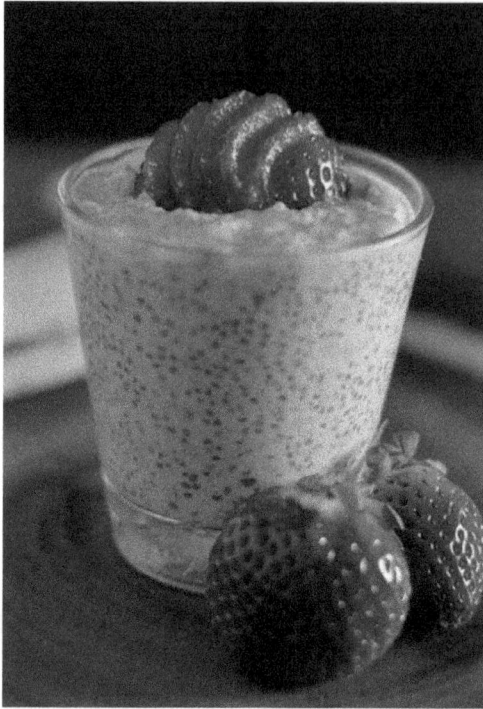

Recipe Time: 30 minutes

Serving Size: 4

Diet Type: Gluten Free, Dairy Free, Soy Free, Vegetarian

Ingredients:

- 1 teaspoon pure vanilla extract
- ¼ cup chia seeds
- ¼ cup shredded coconut, unsweetened
- ¾ cup water

- ¾ cup unsweetened almond milk
- 2 tablespoons raw honey
- ½ cup strawberries, sliced

Cooking Instructions:

1. In a bowl (medium size), whisk the water, milk, and vanilla.
2. Add the chia seeds, and mix well. Cover the bowl, and refrigerate for 30 minutes or overnight.
3. Mix in the coconut and honey.
4. Add the porridge into serving bowls. Serve topped with the strawberries.

Nutritional Values (Per Serving):

Calories 123, Fat 7g, Carbohydrates 14g, Fiber 5g, Protein 2g

Pepper Egg Breakfast

Recipe Time: 5 minutes

Serving Size: 2

Diet Type: Gluten Free, Dairy Free, Soy Free, Nut Free

Ingredients:

- A pinch of garlic powder
- A pinch of (ground) black pepper and salt
- 1 tablespoon olive oil
- ½ cup yellow onions, chopped
- ½ cup red bell pepper, chopped
- 2 eggs

Cooking Instructions:

1. In a skillet (you can also use a saucepan); heat the oil over medium stove flame.
2. Add the onions, stir the mixture and cook while stirring for about 2-3 minutes until softened.
3. Add the bell pepper, garlic powder, salt and pepper, stir and cook for 2-3 minutes more.
4. Add the eggs, stir-cook until the eggs are cooked well.
5. Serve warm.

Nutritional Values (Per Serving):

Calories 216, Fat 6g, Carbohydrates 14g, Fiber 7g, Protein 11g

Hemp Chia Porridge

Recipe Time: 15 minutes

Serving Size: 2

Diet Type: Gluten Free, Dairy Free, Soy Free, Vegan, Vegetarian

Ingredients:

- 2 tablespoons chia seeds
- 1 cup almond milk
- ¼ cup coconut milk
- ¼ cup walnuts, chopped and toasted
- 2 tablespoons hemp seeds, toasted
- ¼ cup coconut, shredded and toasted
- 1 tablespoon coconut oil
- ¼ cup almond butter
- ½ teaspoon turmeric powder
- A pinch of black pepper

Cooking Instructions:

1. In a skillet (you can also use a saucepan); heat the milks over medium stove flame.
2. Add the walnuts, seeds, coconut, turmeric, black pepper; stir-cook for 4-5 minutes.

3. Add the coconut oil and the almond butter, stir the mix and cool down for 5 minutes.

4. Serve and enjoy.

Nutritional Values (Per Serving):

Calories 148, Fat 11g, Carbohydrates 16g, Fiber 6g, Protein 11g

Kale Pistachio Smoothie

Recipe Time: 5 minutes

Serving Size: 2

Diet Type: Gluten Free, Dairy Free, Soy Free, Vegan, Vegetarian

Ingredients:

- 2 frozen bananas, cut into chunks
- ½ cup shelled pistachios
- 1 cup almond milk, unsweetened
- 1 cup shredded kale
- 2 tablespoons pure maple syrup
- 1 teaspoon pure vanilla extract
- 3-4 ice cubes (optional)

Cooking Instructions:

1. Take a high-speed blender (you can also use a food processor) and open top lid.
2. Add the milk and other ingredients. Ice cubes are optional to add (add them if you like your smoothie chilled.)
3. Blend the ingredients over high speed to make a smoothie like texture.
4. Add the blended mixture in glasses and enjoy the fresh smoothie.

Nutritional Values (Per Serving):

Calories 278, Fat 4g, Carbohydrates 41g, Fiber 5g, Protein 6g

Mint Summer Smoothie

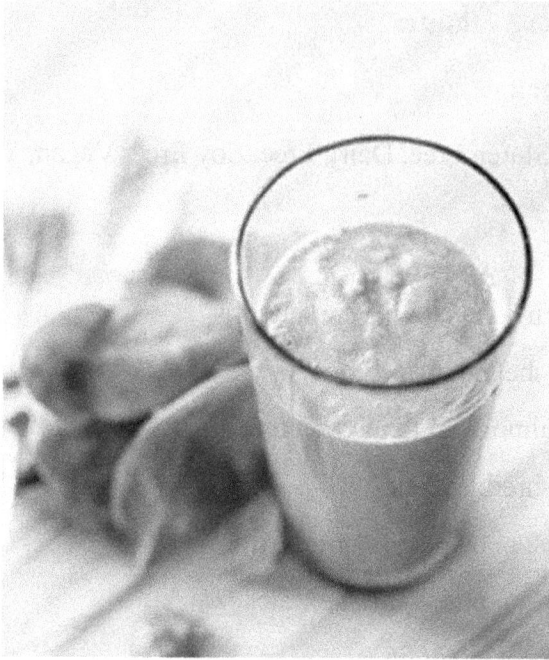

Recipe Time: 5 minutes

Serving Size: 2

Diet Type: Gluten Free, Dairy Free, Soy Free, Nut Free, Vegetarian

Ingredients:

- 1 banana, cut into chunks
- ½ avocado
- 1 cup coconut milk
- 1 cup fresh spinach leaves

- ½ English cucumber, cut into chunks

- 2 tablespoons chopped fresh mint

- 1 tablespoon lemon juice

- 1 tablespoon raw honey

- 3-4 ice cubes (optional)

Cooking Instructions:

1. Take a high-speed blender (you can also use a food processor) and open top lid.

2. Add the milk and other ingredients. Ice cubes are optional to add (add them if you like your smoothie chilled.)

3. Blend the ingredients over high speed to make a smoothie like texture.

4. Add the blended mixture in glasses and enjoy the fresh smoothie.

Nutritional Values (Per Serving):

Calories 384, Fat 21g, Carbohydrates 32g, Fiber 9g, Protein 6g

Fig Yogurt Smoothie

Recipe Time: 5 minutes

Serving Size: 2

Diet Type: Gluten Free, Dairy Free, Soy Free, Vegetarian

Ingredients:

- 1 cup plain whole-milk yogurt
- 1 cup almond milk
- 6-7 whole figs, halved
- 1 banana, cut into chunks
- 1 tablespoon almond butter (optional)
- 1 teaspoon ground flaxseed
- 1 teaspoon raw honey
- Ice cubes (optional)

Cooking Instructions:

1. Take a high-speed blender (you can also use a food processor) and open top lid.
2. Add the milk, yogurt and other ingredients. Ice cubes are optional to add (add them if you like your smoothie chilled.)
3. Blend the ingredients over high speed to make a smoothie like texture.

4. Add the blended mixture in glasses and enjoy the fresh smoothie.

Nutritional Values (Per Serving):

Calories 258, Fat 2g, Carbohydrates 48g, Fiber 9g, Protein 8g

Avocado Cocoa Smoothie

Recipe Time: 5 minutes

Serving Size: 2

Diet Type: Gluten Free, Dairy Free, Soy Free, Vegetarian

Ingredients:

- ½ avocado, pitted and halved
- ½ banana, cut into chunks
- 1 cup unsweetened almond milk
- 1 cup shredded kale
- 1 tablespoon coconut oil
- 1 tablespoon raw honey
- 1 teaspoon pure vanilla extract
- 2 tablespoons cocoa powder
- 4 ice cubes

Cooking Instructions:

1. Take a high-speed blender (you can also use a food processor) and open top lid.
2. Add the milk and other ingredients. Ice cubes are optional to add (add them if you like your smoothie chilled.)

3. Blend the ingredients over high speed to make a smoothie like texture.

4. Add the blended mixture in glasses and enjoy the fresh smoothie.

Nutritional Values (Per Serving):

Calories 286, Fat 19g, Carbohydrates 25g, Fiber 5g, Protein 3g

Pumpkin Cinnamon Smoothie

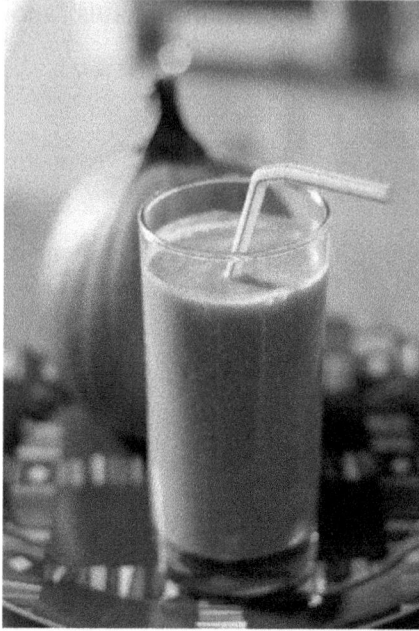

Recipe Time: 5 minutes

Serving Size: 2

Diet Type: Gluten Free, Dairy Free, Soy Free, Vegan, Vegetarian

Ingredients:

- 1 tablespoon maple syrup

- 1 teaspoon (shredded or grated) ginger

- 1 cup unsweetened almond milk

- 1 cup pumpkin purée

- ¼ teaspoon ground cinnamon

- ⅛ teaspoon ground nutmeg

- Pinch ground cloves

- Pinch ground cardamom

- 4 ice cubes

Cooking Instructions:

1. Take a high-speed blender (you can also use a food processor) and open top lid.

2. Add the milk and other ingredients. Ice cubes are optional to add (add them if you like your smoothie chilled.)

3. Blend the ingredients over high speed to make a smoothie like texture.

4. Add the blended mixture in glasses and enjoy the fresh smoothie.

Nutritional Values (Per Serving):

Calories 84, Fat 2g, Carbohydrates 17g, Fiber 4g, Protein 2g

Carrot Pineapple Juice

Recipe Time: 5 minutes

Serving Size: 2

Diet Type: Gluten Free, Dairy Free, Soy Free, Nut Free, Vegan, Vegetarian

Ingredients:

- 8 carrots, peeled and chopped
- 3 cups chopped fresh pineapple
- ¼ cup water
- 1 (1-inch) piece peeled ginger
- Ice cubes, for serving

Cooking Instructions:

1. Take a high-speed blender (you can also use a food processor) and open top lid.
2. Add the milk and other ingredients.
3. Blend the ingredients over high speed to make a smooth mix.
4. Strain the mixture using a cheesecloth in a large bowl. Squeeze through the cheesecloth.
5. Pour the strained mixture in glasses, add the ice cubes (optional) and enjoy the fresh juice.

Nutritional Values (Per Serving):

Calories 124, Fat 1g, Carbohydrates 38g, Fiber 2g, Protein 3g

Cherry Beet Smoothie

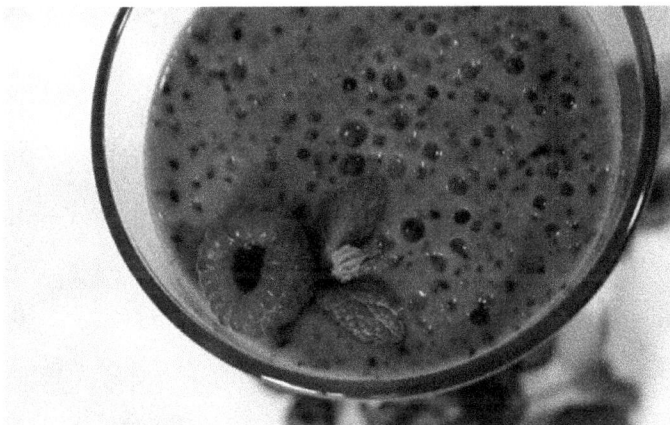

Recipe Time: 5 minutes

Serving Size: 2

Diet Type: Gluten Free, Dairy Free, Soy Free, Vegan, Vegetarian

Ingredients:

- ½ banana, cut into chunks
- ½ cup cherries, pitted
- 10 ounces almond milk
- 2 beets, peeled and cut into small chunks
- 1 tablespoon almond butter
- 3-4 ice cubes (optional)

Cooking Instructions:

1. Take a high-speed blender (you can also use a food processor) and open top lid.

2. Add the milk and other ingredients. Ice cubes are optional to add (add them if you like your smoothie chilled.)

3. Blend the ingredients over high speed to make a smoothie like texture.

4. Add the blended mixture in glasses and enjoy the fresh smoothie.

Nutritional Values (Per Serving):

Calories 156, Fat 5g, Carbohydrates 12g, Fiber 5g, Protein 6g

Pineapple Lush Red Smoothie

Recipe Time: 5 minutes

Serving Size: 2

Diet Type: Gluten Free, Dairy Free, Soy Free, Nut Free, Vegan, Vegetarian

Ingredients:

- 1 banana, cut into chunks
- ½ cup fresh raspberries
- 1 cup coconut water
- ½ cup unsweetened pineapple juice
- ½ cup unsweetened shredded coconut
- 3-4 ice cubes

Cooking Instructions:

1. Take a high-speed blender (you can also use a food processor) and open top lid.
2. Add the coconut water and other ingredients. Ice cubes are optional to add (add them if you like your smoothie chilled.)
3. Blend the ingredients over high speed to make a smoothie like texture.
4. Add the blended mixture in glasses and enjoy the fresh smoothie.

Nutritional Values (Per Serving):

Calories 214, Fat 9g, Carbohydrates 28g, Fiber 7g, Protein 3g

Appetizers
&
Sides

Potato Zucchini Appetizers

Recipe Time: 30 minutes

Serving Size: 4

Diet Type: Gluten Free, Dairy Free, Soy Free, Nut Free, Vegan, Vegetarian

Ingredients:

- 1 yellow bell pepper, diced into small bite size
- 2 zucchini, diced into small bite size
- 1 red bell pepper, diced into small bite size
- 1 red onion, diced into small bite size
- 1 sweet potato, diced into small bite size
- 4 garlic cloves
- ¼ cup extra-virgin olive oil
- 1 teaspoon salt

Cooking Instructions:

1. Preheat an oven to 450°F. Line a baking sheet with a foil.
2. In a mixing bowl, combine the zucchini, red bell pepper, yellow bell pepper, onion, olive oil, sweet potato, garlic, and salt.
3. Arrange evenly on the sheet.
4. Bake for 25 minutes, stirring halfway through. Serve warm.

Nutritional Values (Per Serving):

Calories 176, Fat 12g, Carbohydrates 16g, Fiber 3g, Protein 2g

Spinach Stuffed Mushrooms

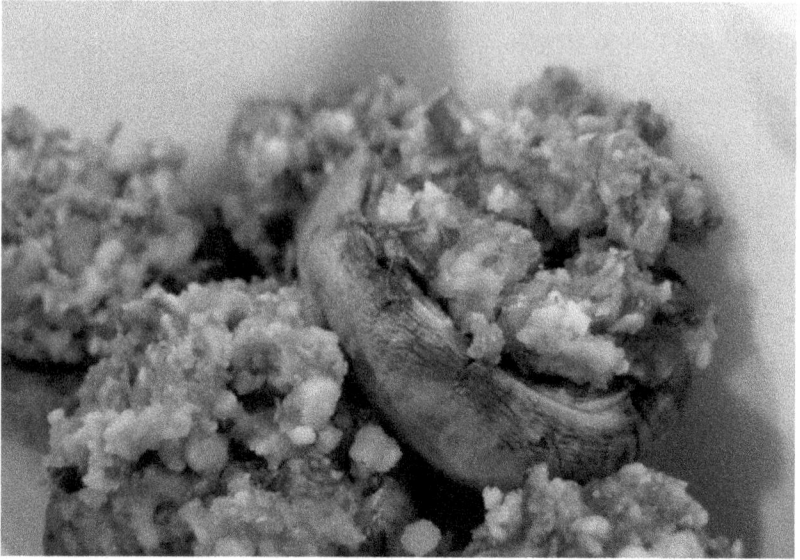

Recipe Time: 35-40 minutes

Serving Size: 12

Diet Type: Gluten Free, Dairy Free, Soy Free, Nut Free, Vegan, Vegetarian

Ingredients:

- 2 pounds button mushrooms, stems reserved
- 3 garlic cloves, minced
- 2 cups spinach, chopped
- 1 tablespoon olive oil
- 2 small red bell peppers, chopped

- 1 small yellow onion, chopped
- (ground) black pepper and salt to the taste
- ¼ cup parsley, chopped

Cooking Instructions:

1. Preheat an oven to 350°F. Line a baking sheet with a foil.
2. In a skillet (you can also use a saucepan); heat the oil over medium stove flame.
3. Add the mushroom, stir and cook for 2 minutes. Set them aside.
4. In the skillet, add the bell peppers, garlic, parsley, spinach, salt, pepper and onion; stir-cook for 5-6 minutes.
5. Stuff each mushroom with the spinach mix.
6. Place them on a lined baking sheet; bake for 20 minutes and serve warm.

Nutritional Values (Per Serving):

Calories 132, Fat 8g, Carbohydrates 9g, Fiber 4g, Protein 9g

Baked Beet Sides

Recipe Time: 30 minutes

Serving Size: 6

Diet Type: Gluten Free, Dairy Free, Soy Free, Nut Free, Vegetarian

Ingredients:

- ½ yellow onion, sliced
- 4 medium golden beets, peeled and diced into small bite size
- 4 medium red beets, peeled and diced into small bite size
- ½ cup apple cider vinegar
- ½ cup extra-virgin olive oil
- 2 tablespoons raw honey
- ¼ teaspoon salt
- Freshly ground black pepper

Cooking Instructions:

1. Preheat an oven to 450°F. Line a baking sheet with a foil.
2. Arrange the beets and onion; drizzle with the vinegar, honey and olive oil.
3. Sprinkle the pepper and salt.
4. Bake for 25 minutes, or until the beets caramelize.
5. Serve warm.

Nutritional Values (Per Serving):

Calories 228, Fat 18g, Carbohydrates 16g, Fiber 3g, Protein 2g

Sesame Bok Choy Side

Recipe Time: 20 minutes

Serving Size: 4

Diet Type: Gluten Free, Dairy Free, Soy Free, Nut Free, Vegan, Vegetarian

Ingredients:

- 1-inch ginger, (shredded or grated)
- 2 tablespoons olive oil
- 3 tablespoons coconut aminos
- A pinch of red pepper flakes
- 4 bok choy heads, cut into quarters
- 2 garlic cloves, minced
- 1 tablespoon sesame seeds, toasted

Cooking Instructions:

1. In a skillet (you can also use a saucepan); heat the oil over medium stove flame.
2. Add the coconut aminos, garlic, pepper flakes and ginger; stir-cook for 4 minutes.
3. Add the bok choy and sesame seeds, toss, cook for 5-6 minutes. Serve warm.

Nutritional Values (Per Serving):

Calories , Fat g, Carbohydrates g, Fiber g, Protein g

Salmon Bites

Recipe Time: 25-30 minutes

Serving Size: 2

Diet Type: Gluten Free, Dairy Free, Soy Free, Nut Free

Ingredients:

- 2 teaspoons garlic powder
- 1 teaspoon onion powder
- 20 ounces canned pineapple pieces
- ½ teaspoon ginger, (shredded or grated)
- 1 tablespoon balsamic vinegar
- 2 salmon fillets, boneless, skinless and cubed
- Black pepper to the taste

Cooking Instructions:

1. Preheat an oven to 375°F. Grease a baking dish with some cooking spray.
2. Place the salmon and pineapple in the dish.
3. Add the ginger, garlic powder, onion powder, black pepper and vinegar, toss the mix.
4. Bake for 20 minutes, divide into bowls and serve.

Nutritional Values (Per Serving):

Calories 198, Fat 2g, Carbohydrates 8g, Fiber 3g, Protein 14g

Garlic Cauliflower

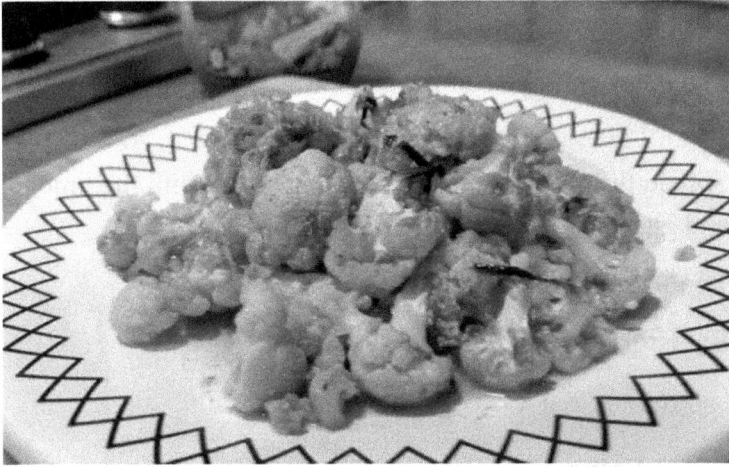

Recipe Time: 15-20 minutes

Serving Size: 4

Diet Type: Gluten Free, Soy Free, Nut Free, Vegetarian

Ingredients:

- ½ teaspoon freshly ground black pepper
- ½ teaspoon garlic powder
- 1½ teaspoons ground cumin
- 1 teaspoon salt
- ½ teaspoon chili powder
- 1 head cauliflower, chopped into bite-size pieces
- 3 tablespoons lime juice
- 3 tablespoons ghee

Cooking Instructions:

1. Preheat an oven to 450°F. Grease a baking dish with some cooking spray.

2. In a bowl, mix the cumin, salt, chili powder, pepper, and garlic powder.

3. Spread the cauliflower in the pan. Drizzle with the lime juice and ghee.

4. Top with the spice mixture and toss to coat.

5. Bake for 15 minutes and serve warm.

Nutritional Values (Per Serving):

Calories 136, Fat 11g, Carbohydrates 9g, Fiber 3g, Protein 4g

Lentil Potato Patties

Recipe Time: 20 minutes

Serving Size: 7-8

Diet Type: Gluten Free, Dairy Free, Soy Free, Vegan, Vegetarian

Ingredients:

- 1 cup canned red lentils, drained and mashed
- 1 sweet potato, (shredded or grated)
- ¼ cup parsley, chopped
- 2 teaspoons ginger, (shredded or grated)
- 1 cup yellow onion, chopped
- 1 cup mushrooms, minced
- 1 tablespoon curry powder
- ¼ cup cilantro, chopped
- 2 tablespoons coconut flour
- 1 tablespoon olive oil

Cooking Instructions:

1. Add the onion, ginger, mushrooms, lentils, potato, curry powder, parsley, cilantro and flour in a bowl.
2. Combine well and prepare patties out of this mix.

3. In a skillet (you can also use a saucepan); heat the oil over medium stove flame.

4. Add the patties and cook for about 5 minutes on each side and serve warm.

Nutritional Values (Per Serving):

Calories 136, Fat 4g, Carbohydrates 7g, Fiber 3g, Protein 8g

Garlic Tomato Sides

Recipe Time: 25 minutes

Serving Size: 6

Diet Type: Gluten Free, Dairy Free, Soy Free, Nut Free, Vegan, Vegetarian

Ingredients:

- 4 garlic cloves, minced
- 1 pound cherry tomatoes, halved
- 1 teaspoon dried basil (optional)
- 2 tablespoons extra-virgin olive oil
- Salt to taste

Cooking Instructions:

1. Preheat an oven to 400°F. Line a baking sheet with a foil.
2. In a bowl, mix the tomatoes, garlic, and basil. Add the olive oil and toss to coat well. Season generously with salt.
3. Add the mix to the sheet.
4. Bake for 15-20 minutes, or until the tomatoes are cooked well.
5. Serve warm.

Nutritional Values (Per Serving):

Calories 47, Fat 0g, Carbohydrates 9g, Fiber 3g, Protein 2g

Awesome Asparagus

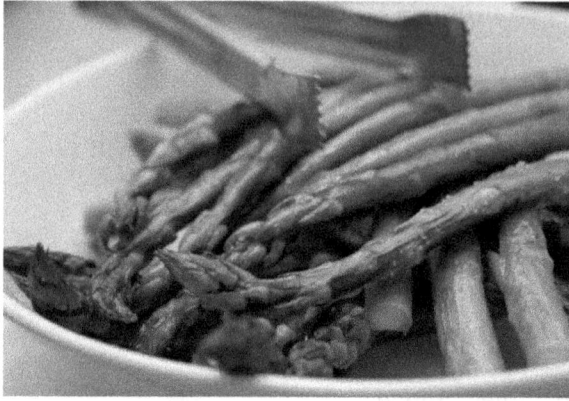

Recipe Time: 25 minutes

Serving Size: 4

Diet Type: Gluten Free, Dairy Free, Soy Free, Nut Free, Vegan, Vegetarian

Ingredients:

- 2 tablespoons shallot, chopped
- 5 tablespoons olive oil
- 4 garlic cloves, minced
- Black pepper to the taste
- 1 ½ teaspoons balsamic vinegar
- 1 ½ pound asparagus, trimmed

Cooking Instructions:

1. Preheat an oven to 450°F. Line a baking sheet with a foil.

2. Spread the asparagus on the sheet.

3. Top with the remaining ingredients and coat well.

4. Bake for 15 minutes and serve warm.

Nutritional Values (Per Serving):

Calories 124, Fat 1g, Carbohydrates 4g, Fiber 2g, Protein 3g

Garlic Kale Sides

Recipe Time: 25 minutes

Serving Size: 4

Diet Type: Gluten Free, Dairy Free, Soy Free, Nut Free, Vegan, Vegetarian

Ingredients:

- 8 cups chopped kale
- 1 tablespoon olive oil
- 3 garlic cloves, crushed
- 1 tablespoon balsamic vinegar
- ½ teaspoon ground nutmeg
- Sea salt to taste

Cooking Instructions:

1. In a skillet (you can also use a saucepan); heat the oil over medium stove flame.
2. Add the garlic, stir the mixture and cook while stirring for about 3-4 minutes until fragrant.
3. Add the kale; stir-cook for about 5-7 minutes, or until wilted.
4. Stir in the balsamic vinegar; sprinkle with nutmeg, and sea salt.
5. Serve warm.

Nutritional Values (Per Serving):

Calories 98, Fat 4g, Carbohydrates 14g, Fiber 3g, Protein 4g

Soups & Stews

Chicken Veggie Dinner Soup

Recipe Time: 55-60 minutes

Serving Size: 6-7

Meal Type: Dinner

Diet Type: Gluten Free, Dairy Free, Soy Free, Nut Free

Ingredients:

- 2 teaspoons minced garlic
- 3 cups shredded fennel
- 3 cups shredded green cabbage
- 1 tablespoon olive oil
- 1 sweet onion, chopped
- 2 carrots, chopped
- 8 cups chicken bone broth
- 2 teaspoons chopped fresh thyme
- 2 cups cooked chicken breast, chopped
- Pinch sea salt to taste

Cooking Instructions:

1. In a cooking pot (you can also use a deep saucepan); heat the oil over medium stove flame.

2. Add the onions, garlic, stir the mixture and cook while stirring for about 2-3 minutes until softened.

3. Stir in the fennel, cabbage, and carrots. Sauté for about 4-5 minutes.

4. Stir in the broth and thyme. Bring the soup to a boil.

5. Reduce the heat to low and simmer the mixture for 25-30 minutes, or until the veggies are tender.

6. Add the chicken and salt. Stir and simmer for about 5 minutes. Serve warm.

Nutritional Values (Per Serving):

Calories 246, Fat 9g, Carbohydrates 16g, Fiber 5g, Protein 24g

Mushroom Lentil Soup

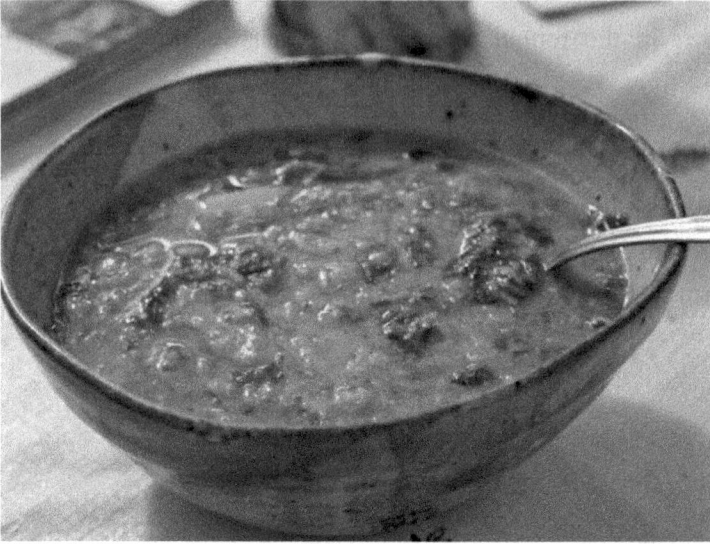

Recipe Time: 30 minutes

Serving Size: 4

Meal Type: Lunch

Diet Type: Gluten Free, Dairy Free, Soy Free, Nut Free, Vegan, Vegetarian

Ingredients:

- 1 medium yellow onion, chopped
- 1 cup white mushrooms, quartered
- 1 1/2 tablespoons coconut oil
- 2 cloves garlic, minced
- 3 cups vegetable broth

- 3 teaspoons miso paste
- 1 cup cooked lentils
- 2 cups kale

Cooking Instructions:

1. In a cooking pot (you can also use a deep saucepan); heat the oil over medium stove flame.
2. Add the garlic, stir the mixture and cook while stirring for about 1 minutes until fragrant.
3. Add the onions and cook for 2-3 minutes until turn soft.
4. Add the mushrooms; stir-cook for another 5 minutes.
5. Add the broth and boil the mixture. Decrease the heat to low flame.
6. Mix in the miso paste and lentils; cook for 5 minute.
7. Stirs in the kale. Let it cook for another 3 minutes.
8. Serve warm.

Nutritional Values (Per Serving):

Calories 294, Fat 4g, Carbohydrates 8g, Fiber 2g, Protein 15g

Pork Chili Stew

Recipe Time: 1 hour 50 minutes

Serving Size: 4-6

Meal Type: Dinner

Diet Type: Gluten Free, Dairy Free, Soy Free, Nut Free

Ingredients:

- 3 tablespoons olive oil
- 3 pounds pork shoulder, cubed
- 2 yellow onions, chopped
- 2 tablespoons garlic, minced
- 2 cups almond flour
- A pinch of (ground) black pepper and salt
- 1 teaspoon chili pepper flakes, dried
- 3 cups chicken stock
- 4 tablespoons sage, chopped
- ¼ cup tomato paste
- ½ teaspoon all-spice

Cooking Instructions:

1. In a bowl (medium size), mix the flour, salt and pepper.

2. Coat the pork in this mix.

3. In a cooking pot (you can also use a deep saucepan); heat the oil over medium stove flame.

4. Add the meat and cook, while stirring, until becomes evenly brown.

5. Transfer it to a bowl.

6. In the pan, add the garlic, onion, sage and pepper flakes and stir-cook for 8 minutes.

7. Add the pork to the pan; mix in the stock, allspice and tomato paste.

8. Stir and cook everything for 80-90 minutes.

9. Divide into serving bowls and serve warm.

Nutritional Values (Per Serving):

Calories 271, Fat 4g, Carbohydrates 11g, Fiber 6g, Protein 18g

Chicken Jalapeno Soup

Recipe Time: 25-30 minutes

Serving Size: 6

Meal Type: Lunch

Diet Type: Gluten Free, Dairy Free, Soy Free, Nut Free

Ingredients:

- 1 tablespoon avocado oil
- 1 jalapeño pepper, seeded and minced
- 6 cups chicken broth
- 1 pound shredded cooked chicken
- 3 garlic cloves, minced
- 1 medium white onion, diced
- 1 (14-ounce) can diced tomatoes with their juice
- 1 (4-ounce) can diced green chiles
- 3 tablespoons lime juice
- ¼ teaspoon cayenne pepper
- Freshly ground black pepper
- 1 teaspoon chili powder
- 1 teaspoon ground cumin
- ½ teaspoon salt
- 1 avocado, pitted and sliced

Cooking Instructions:

1. In a cooking pot (you can also use a deep saucepan); heat the oil over medium stove flame.

2. Add the garlic, onion, and jalapeño pepper; sauté for 4-5 minutes.

3. Add the broth, chicken, tomatoes, chiles, lime juice, chili powder, cumin, salt, cayenne pepper, and black pepper.

4. Stir the mix and bring to a simmer; cook for 10 minutes.

5. Add in serving bowls and too with the slices of avocado and cilantro.

Nutritional Values (Per Serving):

Calories 274, Fat 7g, Carbohydrates 12g, Fiber 4g, Protein 30g

Broccoli Potato Soup

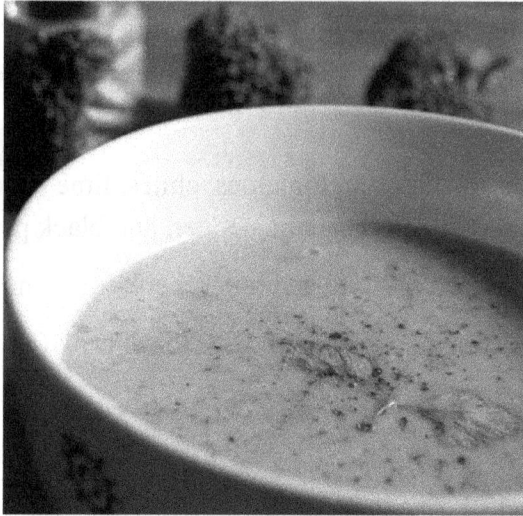

Recipe Time: 40-45 minutes

Serving Size: 6

Meal Type: Lunch

Diet Type: Gluten Free, Dairy Free, Soy Free, Nut Free

Ingredients:

- 1 cup sliced onion
- 2 teaspoons minced garlic
- 1 tablespoon olive oil
- 1 sweet onion, chopped
- 1 sweet potato, peeled and roughly chopped
- 1 teaspoon ground nutmeg

- 8 cups chicken bone broth

- 3 heads broccoli, cut into florets

- ½ cup coconut cream

- Sea salt to taste

Cooking Instructions:

1. In a cooking pot (you can also use a deep saucepan); heat the oil over medium stove flame.

2. Add the onions, garlic, stir the mixture and cook while stirring for about 2-3 minutes until softened.

3. Stir in the broth, broccoli, sweet potato, and nutmeg.

4. Bring it to a boil. Reduce flame to low and simmer for 25-30 minutes, or until the vegetables are tender.

5. Purée the soup in a blender until smooth.

6. Whisk in the cream and season with sea salt. Serve warm.

Nutritional Values (Per Serving):

Calories 184, Fat 9g, Carbohydrates 18g, Fiber 6g, Protein 14g

Tuna Potato Stew

Recipe Time: 40 minutes

Serving Size: 4

Meal Type: Dinner

Diet Type: Gluten Free, Dairy Free, Soy Free, Nut Free

Ingredients:

- 1 teaspoon dried chili
- ¼ pint chicken stock
- 1 yellow onion, chopped
- 1 tablespoon olive oil
- 1 garlic clove, minced
- 14 ounces canned tomatoes, chopped
- 3 sweet potatoes, cubed
- 1 teaspoon sweet paprika
- 2 tuna fillets, flaked
- 1 red pepper, chopped
- 1 tablespoon coriander, chopped

Cooking Instructions:

1. In a cooking pot (you can also use a deep saucepan); heat the oil over medium stove flame.

2. Add the onions, stir the mixture and cook while stirring for about 3-4 minutes until softened.

3. Add the chili and garlic, stir-cook for 1 minute.

4. Add the stock, tomatoes, potatoes, paprika and red pepper, stir the mix.

5. Simmer and cook for 20 minutes over medium flame.

6. Add the tuna, cook for 8-10 minutes.

7. Add into serving bowls, sprinkle coriander on top and serve warm.

Nutritional Values (Per Serving):

Calories 224, Fat 4g, Carbohydrates 16g, Fiber 7g, Protein 7g

Fish Shrimp Soup

Recipe Time: 40 minutes

Serving Size: 6

Meal Type: Dinner

Diet Type: Gluten Free, Dairy Free, Soy Free, Nut Free

Ingredients:

- 2 stalks celery, chopped
- 1 tablespoon olive oil
- 1 sweet onion, chopped
- 2 teaspoons minced garlic
- 2 carrots, diced
- ½ teaspoon ground cumin
- ½ teaspoon ground coriander
- 1 pound haddock, cut into small bite size
- 6 cups chicken bone broth
- 2 cups cubed sweet potato
- ½ pound peeled and deveined shrimp, chopped
- 1 cup chopped spinach
- 2 tablespoons chopped fresh cilantro

Cooking Instructions:

1. In a cooking pot (you can also use a deep saucepan); heat the oil over medium stove flame.

2. Add the onions, garlic, celery, stir the mixture and cook while stirring for about 2-3 minutes until softened.

3. Stir in the broth, sweet potato, carrots, cumin, and coriander.

4. Boil the mix. Reduce flame to low and simmer for about 10 minutes, or until the vegetables are tender.

5. Stir in the haddock and shrimp. Simmer the mix for 8-10 minutes more. Stir in the spinach and simmer for 2 minutes.

6. Add in serving bowls and top with the cilantro.

Nutritional Values (Per Serving):

Calories 244, Fat 8g, Carbohydrates 18g, Fiber 3g, Protein 26g

Yogurt Tomato Soup

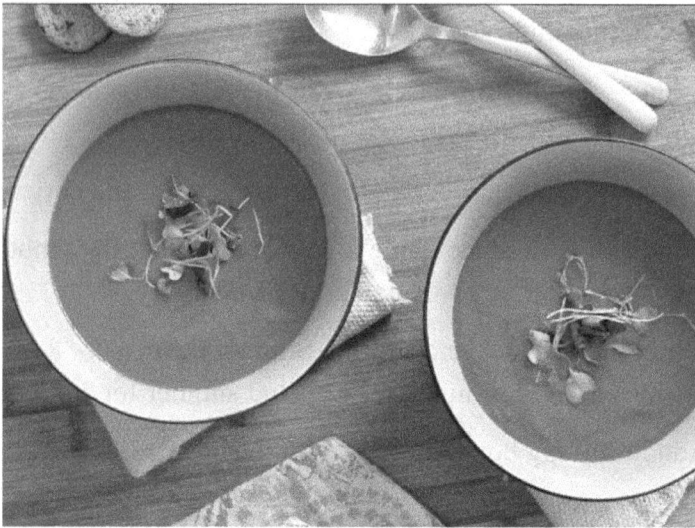

Recipe Time: 25-30 minutes

Serving Size: 6

Meal Type: Lunch

Diet Type: Gluten Free, Soy Free, Nut Free, Vegetarian

Ingredients:

- 1 teaspoon dried basil
- 1 teaspoon dried oregano
- ⅛ teaspoon freshly ground black pepper
- ⅛ teaspoon dried thyme
- ½ teaspoon salt

- ¼ teaspoon chili powder

- 1 tablespoon ghee

- 1 small onion, chopped

- 3 garlic cloves, chopped

- 2 (14-ounce) cans diced tomatoes with their juice

- 2 cups vegetable broth

- ¼ cup tomato paste

- ½ cup plain whole-milk yogurt

Cooking Instructions:

1. In a cooking pot (you can also use a deep saucepan); heat the oil over medium stove flame.

2. Add the onions, garlic, stir the mixture and cook while stirring for about 4-5 minutes until softened.

3. Stir in the basil, oregano, salt, chili powder, pepper, and thyme.

4. Add the tomatoes, broth, and tomato paste; combine well.

5. Bring to a simmer, turn flame to low, and cook for 8-10 minutes.

6. Puree the mix in a blender and add the yogurt. Blend for 1 minute more.

7. Serve warm.

Nutritional Values (Per Serving):

Calories 152, Fat 6g, Carbohydrates 26g, Fiber 12g, Protein 8g

Artichoke Chicken Stew

Recipe Time: 65 minutes

Serving Size: 7-8

Meal Type: Dinner

Diet Type: Gluten Free, Dairy Free, Soy Free, Nut Free

Ingredients:

- 5 garlic cloves, minced
- 2 tablespoons olive oil
- 2 yellow onions, chopped
- 2 pounds chicken thighs, skinless, boneless and chopped
- 1 tablespoon maple syrup
- 2 cups vegetable stock
- 16 ounces canned artichoke hearts, drained and chopped
- A pinch of sea (ground) black pepper and salt
- 2 tablespoons cilantro, chopped

Cooking Instructions:

1. In a cooking pot (you can also use a deep saucepan); heat 1 tablespoon oil over medium stove flame.
2. Add the chicken, and cook, while stirring, until becomes evenly brown.

3. Transfer to a bowl (medium size).

4. In the pan heat the remaining oil, add the garlic and onion, stir and cook for 1 minute.

5. Add the stock, maple syrup, artichokes, salt and pepper, stir the mix.

6. Simmer and cook for 3-4 minutes.

7. Add the chicken to the pot, stir the mix.

8. Cover the pot, reduce flame to low, cook for 45 minutes.

9. Mix in the cilantro and serve warm.

Nutritional Values (Per Serving):

Calories 207, Fat 4g, Carbohydrates 11g, Fiber 4g, Protein 21g

Shrimp Scallops Stew

Recipe Time: 30 minutes

Serving Size: 4

Meal Type: Dinner

Diet Type: Gluten Free, Dairy Free, Soy Free, Nut Free

Ingredients:

- 1 teaspoon jalapeno, chopped
- 2 teaspoons garlic, chopped
- 2 leeks, chopped
- 2 tablespoons olive oil
- 1 carrot, chopped
- 1 teaspoon cumin, ground
- A pinch of (ground) black pepper and salt
- ¼ teaspoon cinnamon powder
- 1 ½ cups tomatoes, chopped
- 1 cup veggie stock
- 1 pound shrimp, peeled and deveined
- 1 pound sea scallops
- 2 tablespoons cilantro, chopped

Cooking Instructions:

1. In a cooking pot (you can also use a deep saucepan); heat the oil over medium stove flame.

2. Add the leek, garlic, stir the mixture and cook while stirring for about 6-7 minutes until softened.

3. Add the jalapeno, salt, pepper, cayenne, carrots, cinnamon and cumin, stir the mix.

4. Cook for 5 minutes. Add the tomatoes, stock, shrimp and scallops, stir the mix.

5. Cook for 5-6 minutes. Add in serving bowls, top with the cilantro and serve warm.

Nutritional Values (Per Serving):

Calories 245, Fat 4g, Carbohydrates 11g, Fiber 5g, Protein 17g

Sprouts Pork Soup

Recipe Time: 25 minutes

Serving Size: 6

Meal Type: Dinner

Diet Type: Gluten Free, Dairy Free, Soy Free, Nut Free

Ingredients:

- 2 tablespoons olive oil
- 5 garlic cloves, minced
- 2 stalks celery, chopped
- ½ pound pork, cubed
- ½ pounds pork, ground
- 3 cups vegetable stock
- 2 scallions, chopped
- Black pepper to the taste
- 1 cup bean sprouts
- 2 tablespoons parsley, chopped
- ½ teaspoon cinnamon powder
- 4 tablespoons coconut aminos
- ½ tablespoon red pepper flakes

Cooking Instructions:

1. In a cooking pot (you can also use a deep saucepan); heat the oil over medium stove flame.

2. Add the pork strips and cook, while stirring, until becomes evenly brown.

3. Transfer to a plate.

4. In the pan, add the garlic, stir and cook for 1-2 minutes.

5. Add the ground pork, pork strips, scallions, celery, stock, black pepper, cinnamon and aminos.

6. Combine well and bring to a boil and cook for 12-15 minutes.

7. Mix in the sprouts, parsley, and pepper flakes, toss well and serve warm.

Nutritional Values (Per Serving):

Calories 296, Fat 4g, Carbohydrates 9g, Fiber 3g, Protein 15g

Chicken White Bean Soup

Recipe Time: 20 minutes

Serving Size: 4

Diet Type: Gluten Free, Dairy Free, Soy Free, Nut Free

Ingredients:

- 2 (4-ounce) cans diced mild green chilies
- 4 cups cooked white beans, drained and rinsed well
- 4 cups chicken broth or vegetable broth
- 1 tablespoon ghee
- 2 small onions, chopped
- 6 garlic cloves, minced
- 1 teaspoon chili powder
- ¼ teaspoon cayenne pepper
- 4 teaspoons ground cumin
- 2 teaspoons dried oregano
- 4 cups shredded cooked chicken
- 2 scallions, (cut into slices)

Cooking Instructions:

1. In a cooking pot (you can also use a deep saucepan); heat the oil over medium stove flame.

2. Add the onions, garlic, stir the mixture and cook while stirring for about 4-5 minutes until softened.

3. Add the chilies, stir-cook for 2 minutes.

4. Stir in the beans, broth, cumin, oregano, chili powder, and cayenne pepper.

5. Simmer the mix and add the chicken. Reduce flame to medium-low, and cook for 8-10 minutes.

6. Top with the scallions and serve warm.

Nutritional Values (Per Serving):

Calories 296, Fat 4g, Carbohydrates 41g, Fiber 12g, Protein 22g

Coconut Avocado Soup

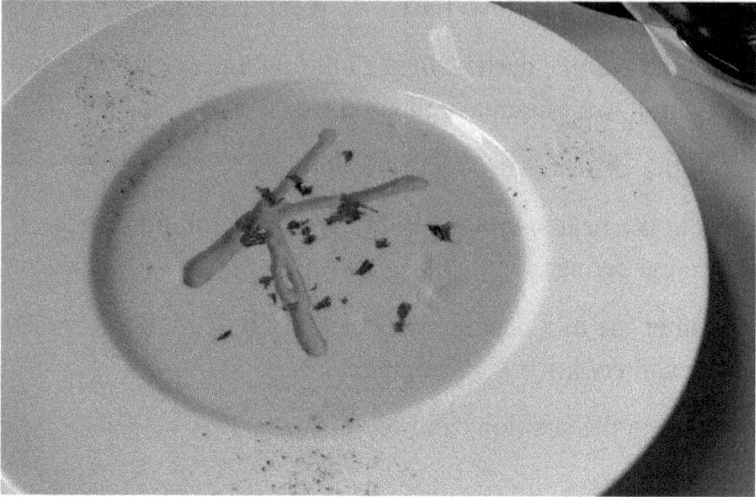

Recipe Time: 15 minutes

Serving Size: 6

Meal Type: Lunch

Diet Type: Gluten Free, Dairy Free, Soy Free, Nut Free, Vegan, Vegetarian

Ingredients:

- 1 tablespoon lemon juice
- 1 garlic clove, crushed
- 1 teaspoon grated ginger
- 3 ripe avocados, peeled and pitted
- ¼ red onion, chopped

- 1 cup chicken bone broth
- ½ teaspoon chopped dill
- 2 cups canned full-fat coconut milk
- Sea salt and ground black pepper to taste

Cooking Instructions:

1. Slice the avocado and set aside.
2. In a blender or food processor, add the avocado, onion, chicken broth, lemon juice, garlic, ginger, and dill. Purée the mixture until very smooth.
3. Transfer in a container. Whisk in the milk. Season with salt and pepper.
4. Chill in your fridge for at least 1 hour.
5. Garnish with the dill sprigs and serve chilled.

Nutritional Values (Per Serving):

Calories 326, Fat 31g, Carbohydrates 14g, Fiber 8g, Protein 4g

Eggplant Pork Stew

Recipe Time: 20 minutes

Serving Size: 4

Meal Type: Dinner

Diet Type: Gluten Free, Dairy Free, Soy Free, Nut Free

Ingredients:

- 4 garlic cloves, minced
- 1 pound pork, ground
- 1 eggplant, cubed
- 2 green onions, chopped
- 2 tablespoons avocado oil
- 14 ounces canned tomatoes, chopped
- (ground) black pepper and salt to the taste
- 1/3 cup basil, chopped
- 2 tablespoons tomato paste
- ¾ cup coconut cream

Cooking Instructions:

1. In a cooking pot (you can also use a deep saucepan); heat the oil over medium stove flame.
2. Add the onions, garlic, stir the mixture and cook while stirring for about 2-3 minutes until softened.
3. Add the beef, stir-cook for 4-5 minutes.

4. Add the eggplant, tomatoes, salt, pepper and basil, stir the mix and cook for 4-5 minutes.

5. Add the tomato paste and cream, stir, cook for 1 minute. Serve warm.

Nutritional Values (Per Serving):

Calories 253, Fat 11g, Carbohydrates 8g, Fiber 1g, Protein 19g

Spinach Mushroom Soup

Recipe Time: 45 minutes

Serving Size: 4

Meal Type: Lunch

Diet Type: Gluten Free, Dairy Free, Soy Free, Nut Free

Ingredients:

- 1 cup sliced mushrooms
- ½ teaspoon fish sauce
- 3 tablespoons miso paste
- 3 cups filtered water
- 3 cups vegetable broth
- 1 cup baby spinach, thoroughly washed
- 4 scallions, (cut into slices)

Cooking Instructions:

1. In a cooking pot (you can also use a deep saucepan); heat the water and broth over medium stove flame.
2. Add the mushrooms, and fish sauce, and boil the mixture. Remove from the heat.
3. In a bowl, mix the miso paste with ½ cup of broth mix. Combine well to dissolve the paste.

4. Add the mix back into the soup. Stir in the spinach and scallions. Serve warm.

Nutritional Values (Per Serving):

Calories 54, Fat 0g, Carbohydrates 9g, Fiber 1g, Protein 2g

Poultry & Chicken

Turkey Green Salad

Recipe Time: 20 minutes

Serving Size: 4

Meal Type: Lunch

Diet Type: Gluten Free, Dairy Free, Soy Free

Ingredients:

Dressing:

- 2 tablespoons balsamic vinegar
- 2 teaspoons Dijon mustard
- ¼ cup olive oil
- 1 teaspoon chopped fresh thyme
- Sea salt to taste

Salad:

- ½ red onion, (cut into slices)
- 4 cups mixed greens
- 1 cup arugula
- 16 ounces cooked turkey breast, chopped
- 3 apricots, pitted and make small pieces
- ½ cup chopped pecans

Cooking Instructions:

1. In a small bowl, whisk the dressing ingredients and set aside.

2. In a salad bowl, add the mixed greens, arugula, and red onion.

3. Top with 3/4 of the dressing.

4. Top with the turkey, apricots, and pecans. Drizzle with the remaining dressing and serve.

Nutritional Values (Per Serving):

Calories 296, Fat 19g, Carbohydrates 12g, Fiber 2g, Protein 21g

Chicken Swiss Salad

Recipe Time: 20 minutes

Serving Size: 6

Meal Type: Lunch

Diet Type: Gluten Free, Dairy Free, Soy Free

Ingredients:

- 4 mini bell peppers, (cut into slices)
- 1 pear, (cut into slices)
- ¼ cup toasted pine nuts
- 2 cups shredded cooked chicken
- 6 cups chopped Swiss chard
- 1 shallot, minced
- ½ cup extra-virgin olive oil
- 2 tablespoons lemon juice
- 2 tablespoons apple cider vinegar
- 1 tablespoon Dijon mustard
- ¼ teaspoon salt

Cooking Instructions:

1. Preheat an oven to 350°F.

2. Wrap the shredded chicken in a piece of aluminum foil; bake for 10 minutes.

3. In a mixing bowl, combine the chard, bell peppers, pear, and nuts.

4. In another bowl, whisk together the shallot, olive oil, lemon juice, vinegar, mustard, and salt.

5. Add the dressing with the nut mix and combine well.

6. Add the baked chicken to the salad. Toss and serve immediately.

Nutritional Values (Per Serving):

Calories 325, Fat 21g, Carbohydrates 9g, Fiber 2g, Protein 14g

Classic Italian Spiced Chicken

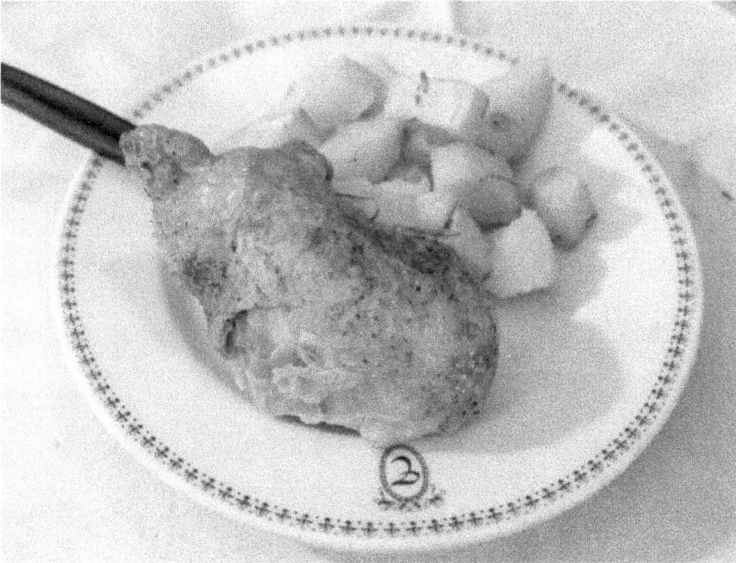

Recipe Time: 70 minutes

Serving Size: 6

Meal Type: Lunch

Diet Type: Gluten Free, Dairy Free, Soy Free, Nut Free

Ingredients:

- 2 tablespoons olive oil

- 1 tablespoon lemon juice

- 1 cup parsley, chopped

- 6 chicken thighs, boneless and skinless

- 2 cups sweet potatoes, cut into wedges

- 2 tablespoons Italian seasoning

Cooking Instructions:

1. Preheat an oven to 450°F. Line a baking sheet with a foil.

2. Add the chicken on a lined sheet; add the potatoes, oil, lemon juice, parsley and seasoning, toss well.

3. Bake the mix for 55-60 minutes until cooked well.

4. Divide between plates and serve.

Nutritional Values (Per Serving):

Calories 236, Fat 7g, Carbohydrates 12g, Fiber 7g, Protein 12g

Chicken Spinach Salad

Recipe Time: 55 minutes

Serving Size: 4

Meal Type: Lunch

Diet Type: Gluten Free, Dairy Free, Soy Free, Nut Free

Ingredients:

- 1 yellow onion, chopped
- 12 ounces mushrooms, chopped
- 2 garlic cloves, minced
- 2 sweet potatoes, baked
- A drizzle of olive oil
- 2 cups baby spinach
- A pinch of salt and cayenne pepper
- ½ teaspoon thyme, dried
- 3 cups chicken, cooked and shredded
- A splash of balsamic vinegar

Cooking Instructions:

1. Cut the potatoes in halves lengthwise; chop into small pieces and add in a bowl (medium size).

2. In a skillet (you can also use a saucepan); heat the oil over medium stove flame.

3. Add the onion, potato pieces, garlic, mushrooms, thyme, chicken, salt and cayenne pepper, toss well.

4. Cook for 8-10 minutes, take off heat.

5. Also add the spinach and vinegar, toss and serve.

Nutritional Values (Per Serving):

Calories 263, Fat 2g, Carbohydrates 17g, Fiber 8g, Protein 11g

Brown Rice Chicken Meal

Recipe Time: 20 minutes

Serving Size: 4

Meal Type: Lunch

Diet Type: Gluten Free, Dairy Free, Soy Free, Nut Free

Ingredients:

- 1 ½ cups brown rice, cooked
- 1 ½ tablespoons maple syrup
- 4 ounces chicken breast boneless, skinless and cut into small pieces
- 1 egg
- 2 egg whites
- 1 cup chicken stock
- 2 tablespoon coconut aminos
- 2 scallions, chopped

Cooking Instructions:

1. In a cooking pot (you can also use a deep saucepan); heat the stock over medium stove flame.
2. Add coconut aminos and sugar, stir the mix and boil it.
3. Add the chicken and toss.
4. In a bowl (medium size), whisk the egg with egg whites.

5. Add it over the chicken mix, add the scallions on top and cook for 3 minutes without stirring.

6. Divide into serving bowls and serve.

Nutritional Values (Per Serving):

Calories 246, Fat 11g, Carbohydrates 13g, Fiber 6g, Protein 9g

Turkey Pepper Patties

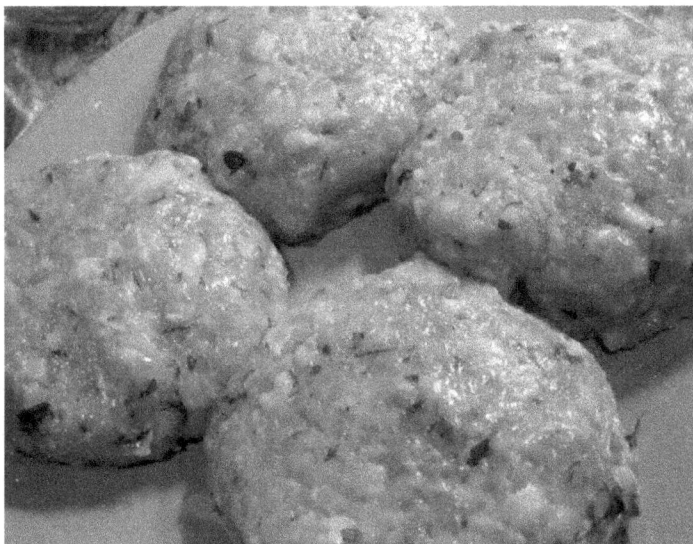

Recipe Time: 20 minutes

Serving Size: 4

Meal Type: Lunch

Diet Type: Gluten Free, Dairy Free, Soy Free, Nut Free

Ingredients:

- 1 pound turkey meat, ground
- 1 small jalapeno pepper, minced
- 2 teaspoons lime juice
- 1 shallot, minced

- 1 tablespoon olive oil

- Zest of 1 lime

- (ground) black pepper and salt to the taste

- 1 teaspoon turmeric powder

Cooking Instructions:

1. In a bowl (medium size), mix the turkey, shallot, jalapeno, lime juice, lime zest, salt, pepper and turmeric.

2. Prepare burger patties from this mix.

3. In a skillet (you can also use a saucepan); heat the oil over medium stove flame.

4. Add the patties and cook them for about 5 minutes on each side.

5. Serve with yogurt dip or green vegetables (optional).

Nutritional Values (Per Serving):

Calories 196, Fat 13g, Carbohydrates 12g, Fiber 5g, Protein 7g

Brussels Chicken Meal

Recipe Time: 20 minutes

Serving Size: 4

Meal Type: Dinner

Diet Type: Gluten Free, Dairy Free, Soy Free

Ingredients:

- 12 ounces Brussels sprouts, shredded
- 1 apple, cored and sliced
- ½ red onion, (cut into slices)
- 1 ½ pounds chicken thighs, skinless and boneless
- 1 tablespoon olive oil
- 2 teaspoons thyme, chopped
- A pinch of (ground) black pepper and salt
- 1 garlic clove, minced
- 2 tablespoons balsamic vinegar
- ¼ cup walnuts, chopped

Cooking Instructions:

1. In a skillet (you can also use a saucepan); heat the oil over medium stove flame.

2. Add the chicken, pepper, salt and thyme; cook, while stirring, until becomes evenly brown.

3. Transfer to a bowl (medium size).

4. In the pan, add the onion, apple, sprouts and garlic, stir-cook for 4-5 minutes.

5. Add the vinegar, cooked chicken, and walnuts, toss, cook for 1-2 minutes.

6. Serve warm.

Nutritional Values (Per Serving):

Calories 223, Fat 4g, Carbohydrates 13g, Fiber 7g, Protein 9g

Broccoli Chicken Light Casserole

Recipe Time: 55 minutes

Serving Size: 4

Meal Type: Lunch

Diet Type: Gluten Free, Dairy Free, Soy Free, Nut Free

Ingredients:

- 8 ounces mushrooms, (cut into slices)
- 3 cups chicken, cooked and shredded
- 4 cups broccoli florets
- 1 yellow onion, chopped
- 2 tablespoons olive oil
- (ground) black pepper and salt to the taste
- 1 cup chicken stock
- ½ teaspoon nutmeg, ground
- 2 eggs

Cooking Instructions:

1. Preheat an oven to 350°F. Grease a baking dish with some cooking spray.
2. In a skillet (you can also use a saucepan); heat the oil over medium stove flame.
3. Add the onions, salt, pepper, mushrooms, stir the mixture and cook while stirring for about 8-10 minutes until softened.

4. Add the mix into a baking dish; mix in the chicken and broccoli

5. In a bowl (medium size), combine the stock, eggs, nutmeg, salt and pepper.

6. Add it over the chicken mix, bake for 40 minutes.

7. Divide between serving plates and serve warm.

Nutritional Values (Per Serving):

Calories 339, Fat 12g, Carbohydrates 13g, Fiber 3g, Protein 16g

Couscous Carrot Chicken

Recipe Time: 30 minutes

Serving Size: 4

Meal Type: Dinner

Diet Type: Dairy Free, Soy Free, Nut Free

Ingredients:

- 1/3 cup roasted pepitas
- 1/3 cup parsley, chopped
- ¼ cup mint, chopped
- 6 ounces couscous, cooked
- 2 teaspoon coconut oil, melted
- 12 ounces baby carrots
- 4 chicken thighs, boneless
- A pinch of (ground) black pepper and salt
- 1 tablespoon lemon juice
- 2 teaspoons lemon zest
- 1 tablespoon olive oil
- 1 garlic clove, minced

Cooking Instructions:

1. Preheat an oven to 450°F. Grease a baking dish with some cooking spray.

2. In a skillet (you can also use a saucepan); heat the oil over medium stove flame.

3. Add the chicken, salt, pepper and cook, while stirring, until becomes evenly brown for 8-10 minutes.

4. Transfer to the baking dish.

5. In the pan, add the carrots and cook for 2-3 minutes.

6. Add the carrots with the chicken; bake for 10 minutes.

7. In a bowl (medium size), mix the couscous, olive oil, salt, pepper, pepitas, parsley, mint, garlic, lemon juice and lemon zest; combine well.

8. Divide the chicken mix between serving plates, add the couscousmix and serve warm.

Nutritional Values (Per Serving):

Calories 264, Fat 4g, Carbohydrates 16g, Fiber 6g, Protein 10g

Turkey Lunch Wraps/Cups

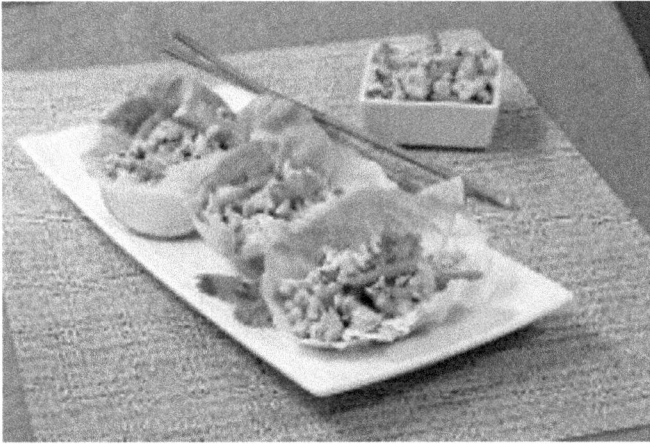

Recipe Time: 25 minutes

Serving Size: 4

Meal Type: Lunch

Diet Type: Gluten Free, Dairy Free, Soy Free, Nut Free

Ingredients:

- 1 pound ground turkey
- 2 tablespoons lime juice
- 2 tablespoons fish sauce
- 2 tablespoons minced cilantro
- 1 tablespoon minced mint (optional)
- 1 tablespoon maple syrup
- 1 small red onion, diced

- 2 garlic cloves, minced

- 4 scallions, (cut into slices)

- ¼ teaspoon red pepper flakes

- 8 small romaine lettuce leaves

Cooking Instructions:

1. In a skillet (you can also use a saucepan); heat the oil over medium stove flame.

2. Add the turkey and cook, while stirring, until becomes evenly brown.

3. Add the onion and garlic, and stir-cook for 8-10 minutes.

4. Remove from the heat.

5. Mix the scallions, lime juice, fish sauce, cilantro, mint, maple syrup, and red pepper flakes; combine well.

6. Add the mix in lettuce leaf. Serve warm.

Nutritional Values (Per Serving):

Calories 153, Fat 2g, Carbohydrates 8g, Fiber 1g, Protein 24g

Spinach Baked Chicken

Recipe Time: 30 minutes

Serving Size: 4

Meal Type: Dinner

Diet Type: Gluten Free, Dairy Free, Soy Free, Nut Free

Ingredients:

- 4 (4-ounce) boneless, skinless chicken breasts
- 1 cup cremini mushrooms, sliced
- ½ red onion, thinly sliced
- ½ cup chopped basil
- 2 tablespoons avocado oil
- 1 pint cherry tomatoes, halved
- 4 garlic cloves, minced
- 2 teaspoons balsamic vinegar
- 1 cup chopped spinach

Cooking Instructions:

1. Preheat an oven to 400°F. Grease a baking dish with some cooking spray.
2. Place the chicken. Brush with the oil.
3. In a bowl (medium size), mix the tomatoes, spinach, mushrooms, red onion, basil, garlic, and vinegar.

4. Top each chicken breast with 1/4th vegetable mixture. Bake for about 18-20 minutes, or until the chicken is cooked well.

5. Serve with the remaining vegetable mix.

Nutritional Values (Per Serving):

Calories 234, Fat 9g, Carbohydrates 8g, Fiber 2g, Protein 27g

Sweet Potato Whole Chicken

Recipe Time: 80-85 minutes

Serving Size: 6

Meal Type: Dinner

Diet Type: Gluten Free, Dairy Free, Soy Free, Nut Free

Ingredients:

- ½ pound sweet potatoes, cubed
- 2 tablespoons olive oil
- 1 whole chicken
- Juice of ½ lemon
- 2 carrots, (cut into slices)
- 3 garlic cloves, minced
- 1 yellow onion, chopped
- 1 rosemary bunch, torn
- A pinch of (ground) black pepper and salt
- 1 thyme bunch, torn

Cooking Instructions:

1. Preheat an oven to 425°F. Grease a baking dish with some cooking spray.
2. Add the chicken in the dish.
3. Mix the oil, rosemary, thyme, salt, pepper, and lemon juice in a bowl. Coat the chicken with it.

135

4. Add the carrots, potatoes and onion in the dish; bake for 60-70 minutes until cooked well.

5. Slice the chicken and serve warm.

Nutritional Values (Per Serving):

Calories 308, Fat 7g, Carbohydrates 16g, Fiber 3g, Protein 22g

Bean Chicken Chili

Recipe Time: 30 minutes

Serving Size: 4

Meal Type: Dinner

Diet Type: Gluten Free, Dairy Free, Soy Free, Nut Free

Ingredients:

- 1 pound chicken, ground
- 30 ounces canned black beans, drained and rinsed
- 28 ounces roasted tomatoes, chopped
- 3 cups butternut squash, cubed
- 1 cup yellow onion, chopped
- 1 ½ tablespoons olive oil
- 2 garlic cloves, minced
- 14 ounces chicken stock
- A pinch of (ground) black pepper and salt

Cooking Instructions:

1. In a skillet (you can also use a saucepan); heat the oil over medium stove flame.
2. Add the garlic, onion, chicken stir the mixture and cook while stirring for about 5-6 minutes until softened.

3. Add the beans, tomatoes, squash, stock, salt and pepper, toss the mix,

4. Simmer and cook for 12-15 minutes.

5. Add into serving bowls and serve warm.

Nutritional Values (Per Serving):

Calories 258, Fat 5g, Carbohydrates 10g, Fiber 4g, Protein 12g

Stuffed Pepper Delight

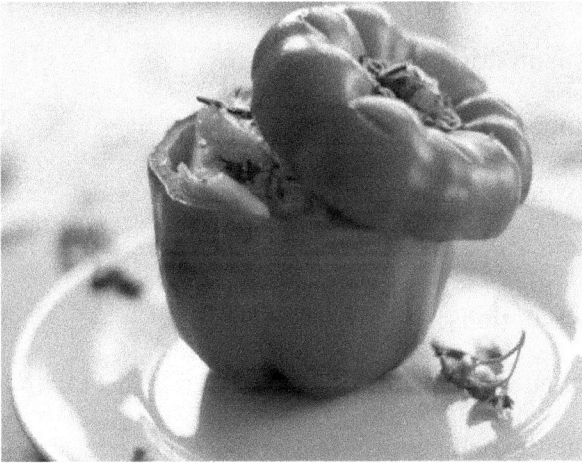

Recipe Time: 20 minutes

Serving Size: 3

Meal Type: Dinner

Diet Type: Gluten Free, Dairy Free, Soy Free, Nut Free

Ingredients:

- 1 small white onion, diced

- 2 garlic cloves, minced

- 1 (16-ounce) can diced tomatoes, drained

- 6 yellow, red or green bell peppers, tops and ribs removed, seeded

- 1 tablespoon avocado or coconut oil

- 1 pound ground turkey

- ½ teaspoon ground cumin
- ½ teaspoon paprika
- ½ teaspoon dried oregano
- ½ teaspoon salt
- Freshly ground black pepper

Cooking Instructions:

1. Preheat an oven to 400°F. Line a baking sheet with a foil.
2. Arrange the bell peppers on the sheet. Drizzle with some oil.
3. Bake for 20 minutes, or until softened.
4. In a skillet (you can also use a saucepan); heat the oil over medium stove flame.
5. Add the turkey and cook, while stirring, until becomes evenly brown for 4-5 minutes.
6. Add the onion and garlic; stir-cook for 8-10 minutes until softened.
7. Stir in the tomatoes, cumin, paprika, oregano, and salt, and season with pepper.
8. Fill the baked peppers with the meat mixture. Serve warm.

Nutritional Values (Per Serving):

Calories 193, Fat 9g, Carbohydrates 12g, Fiber 4g, Protein 14g

Orange Peas Chicken

Recipe Time: 20 minutes

Serving Size: 4

Meal Type: Dinner

Diet Type: Dairy Free, Nut Free

Ingredients:

- 1 red onion, (cut into slices)
- 2 cups sugar snap peas
- 2 garlic cloves, minced
- 1 ¼ pounds chicken breast, skinless, boneless and sliced
- 3 tablespoons coconut flour
- 2 tablespoons olive oil
- 2 tablespoons rice vinegar
- 1 tablespoon sesame seeds, toasted
- ½ cup teriyaki sauce
- 1 tablespoon sesame oil
- 2 oranges, peeled and sliced
- 1 tablespoon cilantro, chopped

Cooking Instructions:

1. In a bowl (medium size), mix the chicken, flour and toss well.

2. In a skillet (you can also use a saucepan); heat the oil over medium stove flame.

3. Add the chicken and cook, while stirring, until becomes evenly brown.

4. Add the garlic and the onion, stir-cook for 1-2 minutes.

5. Add the peas and cook for another 2 minutes.

6. Add the sauce, sesame oil, vinegar, sesame seeds, oranges and cilantro; stir-cook for 1-2 minutes.

7. Add the mix in serving plates and serve.

Nutritional Values (Per Serving):

Calories 287, Fat 3g, Carbohydrates 15g, Fiber 6g, Protein 13g

Herbed Broccoli Chicken

Recipe Time: 40-45 minutes

Serving Size: 4

Meal Type: Dinner

Diet Type: Gluten Free, Dairy Free, Soy Free, Nut Free

Ingredients:

- 2 teaspoons mustard
- 3 tablespoons olive oil
- 1 ½ tablespoons rosemary, chopped
- 2 tablespoons parsley, chopped
- 1 garlic clove, minced
- A pinch of (ground) black pepper and salt
- 1 broccoli head, florets separated
- 1 red onion, cut into wedges
- Juice of 1 lemon
- 4 chicken breasts, skin-on and bone-in
- ½ teaspoon red pepper, crushed

Cooking Instructions:

1. Preheat an oven to 425°F.
2. In a baking dish, mix the chicken with half of the oil, lemon juice, parsley, garlic, rosemary and mustard.
3. Coat well and bake for 30 minutes and divide between serving plates.

4. Line a baking sheet with a foil. Spread the broccoli florets, drizzle the rest of the oil over. Add the red onion and crushed pepper, toss gently.

5. Bake for 15 minutes, add next to the chicken and serve.

Nutritional Values (Per Serving):

Calories 268, Fat 13g, Carbohydrates 15g, Fiber 6g, Protein 27g

Pork, Beef & Lamb

Beef Yogurt Meatballs

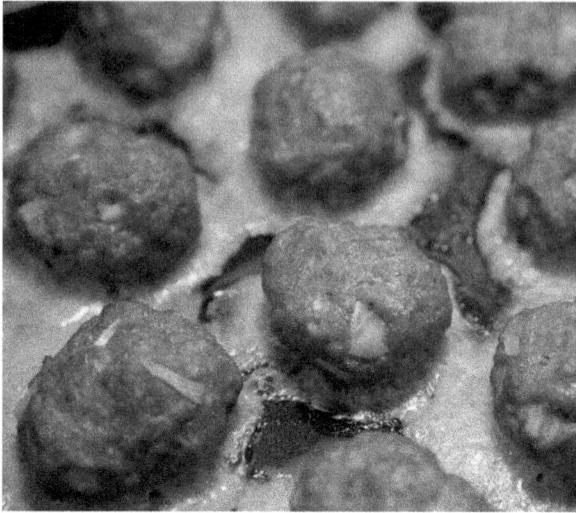

Recipe Time: 60 minutes

Serving Size: 4

Meal Type: Lunch

Diet Type: Gluten Free, Soy Free, Nut Free

Ingredients:

- 2/3 cup plain Greek yogurt
- 1 teaspoon honey
- 1 small sweet potato
- 3 garlic cloves, unpeeled
- 1 small onion, chopped finely
- 1 egg
- (ground) black pepper and salt, to taste, to taste

- ½ pound grass-fed ground beef
- 1 teaspoon ground coriander
- 1 teaspoon ground cumin
- ½ teaspoon cayenne pepper
- 1 tablespoon olive oil

Cooking Instructions:

1. Cook the potatoes to boiling water in a cooking pot for 25-30 minutes then drain.

2. Peel and mash them. Set aside in the large bowl.

3. In a skillet (you can also use a saucepan); heat the olive oil over medium stove flame.

4. Add the garlic, stir the mixture and cook while stirring for about 8-10 minutes until softened.

5. Add the cloves to the food processor or blender.

6. Add the yogurt, honey, salt, and black pepper.

7. Puree the mix until smooth and set aside.

8. Add the egg, ground beef, onion, salt, and spices with the potato bowl. Combine and prepare small meatballs out of this mixture.

9. Take a deep pan and heat oil in it.

10. Add the meatballs in batches and fry for 15-20 minutes until golden brown. Serve with the garlic yogurt.

Nutritional Values (Per Serving):

Calories 276, Fat 14g, Carbohydrates 28g, Fiber 3g, Protein 18g

Lamb Garlic Kebabs with Greens/Rice

Recipe Time: 20-25 minutes

Serving Size: 2-3

Meal Type: Lunch

Diet Type: Gluten Free, Dairy Free, Soy Free, Nut Free

Ingredients:

- 1 tablespoon dried oregano

- 2 teaspoons minced garlic

- 2 tablespoons olive oil

- 2 tablespoons apple cider vinegar

- ½ teaspoon sea salt

- 1 pound lamb shoulder, cut into 1-inch cubes

Cooking Instructions:

1. In a mixing bowl, combine the olive oil, cider vinegar, oregano, garlic, and sea salt.

2. Mix in the lamb. Cover and refrigerate it for 1-2 hour to marinate.

3. Preheat your broiler. Arrange a rack on higher side.

4. Take 8 wooden skewers, thread 4 or 5 pieces of lamb on each and arrange them on a baking sheet.

5. Broil for about 12-15 minutes total, turn in between, until browned evenly.

6. Serve with mixed greens or cooked rice (optional).

Nutritional Values (Per Serving):

Calories 426, Fat 26g, Carbohydrates 3g, Fiber 1g, Protein 54g

Cinnamon Pork Chops

Recipe Time: 35 minutes

Serving Size: 4

Meal Type: Lunch

Diet Type: Gluten Free, Dairy Free, Soy Free, Nut Free

Ingredients:

- 4 pork chops

- ½ teaspoon cinnamon powder

- ½ teaspoon sweet paprika

- A drizzle of olive oil

- A pinch of (ground) black pepper and salt

Cooking Instructions:

1. In a bowl (medium size), coat the pork chops with salt, pepper, oil, cinnamon and paprika.

2. Heat up a grill over medium-high flame.

3. Cook the pork chops for 10-15 minutes on each side, until cook well.

4. Serve with a side salad.

Nutritional Values (Per Serving):

Calories 248, Fat 6g, Carbohydrates 15g, Fiber 7g, Protein 17g

Mustard Lamb Lunch

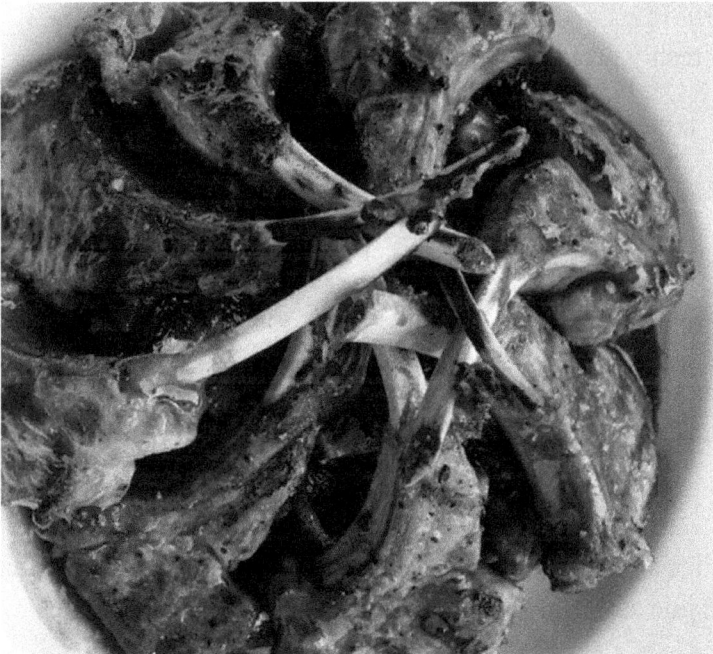

Recipe Time: 45 minutes

Serving Size: 4

Meal Type: Lunch

Diet Type: Gluten Free, Dairy Free, Soy Free, Nut Free

Ingredients:

- 2 (8-rib) lamb racks, patted dry

- ¼ cup Dijon mustard

- 2 tablespoons chopped fresh thyme

- 1 tablespoon chopped fresh rosemary

- Freshly ground black pepper and salt to taste

- 1 tablespoon olive oil

Cooking Instructions:

1. Preheat an oven to 425°F.

2. In a mixing bowl, stir together the mustard, thyme, and rosemary.

3. Coat the lamb racks with sea salt and pepper.

4. Place a large ovenproof skillet over medium-high cooking flame and heat the olive oil.

5. Add the lamb rack; stir-cook for about 2 minutes per side, turning once.

6. Take it off the heat and top with the mustard mix.

7. Bake for 30 minutes or until cooks well.

8. Remove the lamb racks and cut into pieces. Serve warm.

Nutritional Values (Per Serving):

Calories 413, Fat 24g, Carbohydrates 2g, Fiber 1g, Protein 52g

Bok Choy Steak Dinner

Recipe Time: 20 minutes

Serving Size: 4

Meal Type: Dinner

Diet Type: Gluten Free, Dairy Free, Soy Free, Nut Free

Ingredients:

- 2 teaspoons avocado oil

- 1 tablespoon sesame oil

- 2 garlic cloves, minced

- 12 ounces flank steak, cut into thin 2-inch strips

- ½ teaspoon salt

- ¼ teaspoon black pepper

- 4 heads baby bok choy, quartered lengthwise

- 1 tablespoon (shredded or grated) peeled fresh ginger

- 1 tablespoon coconut sugar or maple syrup

- 3 tablespoons coconut aminos

- 2 tablespoons rice vinegar

- ¼ teaspoon red pepper flakes (optional)

Cooking Instructions:

1. Season the with the salt and pepper.

2. In a skillet (you can also use a saucepan); heat the oil over medium stove flame.

3. Add the steak and cook, while stirring, until becomes evenly brown.

4. Transfer to a plate.

5. In the skillet, add the sesame oil and garlic. Stir-cook for 2-3 minutes.

6. Stir in the vinegar, ginger, coconut sugar, bok choy, coconut aminos, and red pepper flakes until well combined.

7. Cover and cook for 2 minutes.

8. Add the steak and toss gently; serve warm.

Nutritional Values (Per Serving):

Calories 246, Fat 13g, Carbohydrates 13g, Fiber 8g, Protein 21g

Apple Pork Raisins

Recipe Time: 40 minutes

Serving Size: 4

Meal Type: Dinner

Diet Type: Gluten Free, Dairy Free, Soy Free

Ingredients:

Salsa:

- ½ teaspoon (shredded or grated) fresh ginger
- 2 apples, peeled, cored, and diced
- 1 teaspoon olive oil
- ¼ cup finely chopped sweet onion
- ½ cup dried raisins
- Pinch sea salt

Chops:

- 4 (4-ounce) boneless center-cut pork chops, trimmed and patted dry
- Freshly ground black pepper and salt to taste
- 1 teaspoon garlic powder
- 1 teaspoon ground cinnamon
- 1 tablespoon olive oil

Cooking Instructions:

1. In a skillet (you can also use a saucepan); heat the oil over medium stove flame.

2. Add the onions, ginger, stir the mixture and cook while stirring for about 2-3 minutes until softened.

3. Stir in the apples and raisins. Sauté for about 4-5 minutes.

4. Season with sea salt and set it aside.

5. Coat the pork chops on both sides with the garlic powder, cinnamon, sea salt, and pepper.

6. In a skillet (you can also use a saucepan); heat the oil over medium stove flame.

7. Add the chops and cook, while stirring, until becomes evenly brown.

8. Serve the chops with the apple salsa.

Nutritional Values (Per Serving):

Calories 384, Fat 27g, Carbohydrates 11g, Fiber 2g, Protein 26g

Avocado Pineapple Pork

Recipe Time: 50 minutes

Serving Size: 4

Meal Type: Dinner

Diet Type: Gluten Free, Dairy Free, Soy Free, Nut Free

Ingredients:

- 1 teaspoon cumin
- 8 ounces canned pineapple, crushed
- 1 tablespoon olive oil
- 1 pound pork, ground
- 1 teaspoon chili powder
- 1 teaspoon garlic powder
- (ground) black pepper and salt to taste
- 1 mango, chopped
- Juice of 1 lime
- 2 avocados, pitted, peeled and chopped
- ¼ cup cilantro, chopped

Cooking Instructions:

1. In a skillet (you can also use a saucepan); heat the oil over medium stove flame.
2. Add the pork and cook, while stirring, until becomes evenly brown.

3. Add the garlic, cumin, chili powder, salt and pepper, stir-cook for 7-8 minutes.

4. Add the pineapple, mango, avocados, lime juice, cilantro, salt and pepper; stir-cook for 5-6 minutes.

5. Divide between serving plates and serve.

Nutritional Values (Per Serving):

Calories 238, Fat 6g, Carbohydrates 12g, Fiber 7g, Protein 17g

Herbed Tomato Chops

Recipe Time: 65-70 minutes

Serving Size: 4

Meal Type: Dinner

Diet Type: Gluten Free, Dairy Free, Soy Free, Nut Free

Ingredients:

- 28 ounces canned tomatoes, chopped

- ¼ cup chicken stock

- 1 cup tomato sauce

- ¼ cup balsamic vinegar

- 2 tablespoons olive oil

- 4 pork chops

- A pinch of (ground) black pepper and salt

- 2 garlic cloves, minced

- 1 yellow onion, chopped

- 1 tablespoon herbs de Provence

- 2 tablespoons parsley, chopped

- 1 tablespoon basil, chopped

Cooking Instructions:

1. In a skillet (you can also use a saucepan); heat the oil over medium stove flame.

2. Add the pork, pepper, salt and cook, while stirring, until becomes evenly brown.

3. Transfer to a serving plate.

4. In a skillet (you can also use a saucepan); heat the oil over medium stove flame.

5. Add the onions, garlic, stir the mixture and cook while stirring for about 8-10 minutes until softened.

6. Add the tomatoes, stock, tomato sauce, vinegar, herbs and parsley, stir-cook for 8-10 minutes.

7. Add the pork and basil, stir, cook for 4-5 minutes more. Add the mix between plates and serve.

Nutritional Values (Per Serving):

Calories 208, Fat 6g, Carbohydrates 9g, Fiber 5g, Protein 18g

Garlic Basil Pork Chops

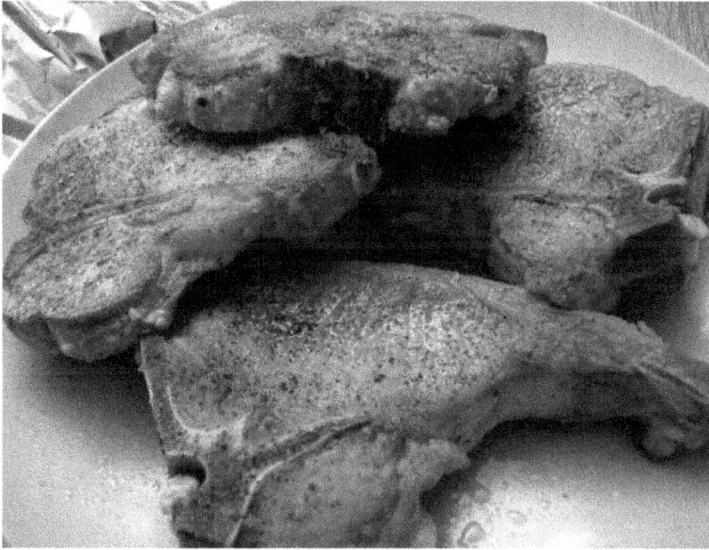

Recipe Time: 20 minutes

Serving Size: 4

Meal Type: Dinner

Diet Type: Gluten Free, Dairy Free, Soy Free, Nut Free

Ingredients:

- 1 cup basil, minced

- 2 tablespoons lemon juice

- 4 pork loin chops

- 2 tablespoons garlic, minced

- 2 tablespoons olive oil

- A pinch of (ground) black pepper and salt

Cooking Instructions:

1. In a bowl (medium size), mix the garlic, oil, basil, lemon juice, salt and pepper. Combine well.

2. Add pork chops and toss well.

3. Place the chops over the preheated grill; cook them for 6 minutes on each side.

4. Add in serving plates and serve warm.

Nutritional Values (Per Serving):

Calories 314, Fat 6g, Carbohydrates 19g, Fiber 6g, Protein 23g

Nutty Pork Steak

Recipe Time: 15 minutes

Serving Size: 4

Meal Type: Dinner

Diet Type: Gluten Free, Dairy Free, Soy Free

Ingredients:

- ¼ cup basil, chopped

- 1 tablespoons garlic, minced

- ¼ cup balsamic vinegar

- 1 pound pork steaks

- 2 tablespoons olive oil

- (ground) black pepper and salt to taste

- 1 teaspoon onion powder

For the pesto:

- ¼ cup olive oil

- ¼ cup pine nuts

- ½ cup bell peppers, roasted

- ½ cup basil, chopped

- 1 garlic clove

- (ground) black pepper and salt to taste

Cooking Instructions:

1. In a bowl (medium size), season the steaks with vinegar, 2 tablespoons oil, basil, garlic, onion, salt and pepper. Add in the fridge for 3-4 hours.

2. Heat your grill over medium-high cooking flame, add the steaks, cook for 4 minutes each side.

3. In your food processor or blender, add the basil with roasted peppers, pine nuts, ¼ cup olive oil, garlic, salt and pepper. Blend to make a smooth mix.

Serve the steaks with the pesto on top.

Nutritional Values (Per Serving):

Calories 276, Fat 7g, Carbohydrates 18g, Fiber 5g, Protein 21g

Beef Bread-Less Meatloaf

Recipe Time: 60 minutes

Serving Size: 4

Meal Type: Dinner

Diet Type: Gluten Free, Dairy Free, Soy Free, Nut Free

Ingredients:

- 1 egg
- 1½ pounds lean ground beef
- ½ cup almond flour
- ½ cup chopped sweet onion
- 1 tablespoon chopped fresh basil
- 1 tablespoon chopped fresh parsley
- 1 teaspoon (shredded or grated) fresh horseradish
- ⅛ teaspoon sea salt

Cooking Instructions:

1. Preheat an oven to 350°F. Grease a loaf pan with some cooking spray.

2. In a mixing bowl, combine the beef, almond flour, onion, egg, basil, parsley, horseradish, and sea salt.

3. Add the meat mixture into the loaf pan.

4. Bake for about 55-60 minutes until cooked through.

5. Remove the pan and serve warm.

Nutritional Values (Per Serving):

Calories 412, Fat 17g, Carbohydrates 5g, Fiber 2g, Protein 53g

Zucchini Jalapeno Pork Meal

Recipe Time: 30 minutes

Serving Size: 4

Meal Type: Dinner

Diet Type: Gluten Free, Dairy Free, Soy Free, Nut Free

Ingredients:

- 3 tablespoons lime juice

- 1 tablespoon olive oil

- 1 jalapeno, halved and seeded

- 3 tomatoes, halved

- 1 red onion, halved

- 4 pork steaks

- 2 zucchinis, (cut into slices)

- ½ cup cilantro, chopped

- 1 garlic clove, minced

- A pinch of(ground) black pepper and salt

Cooking Instructions:

1. Preheat an oven to 475°F. Grease a roasting pan with some cooking spray.

2. Add the tomatoes, zucchini, jalapeno and onion in the pan, and bake for 10 minutes.

3. In a bowl (medium size), mix the olive oil with garlic, cilantro, lime juice, black pepper and salt, whisk.

4. Add to the pan, toss well and divide between serving plates.

5. In a skillet (you can also use a saucepan); coat with some cooking spray. .

6. Add the steak, salt, pepper and cook, while stirring, until becomes evenly brown.

7. Add it with the veggies and serve.

Nutritional Values (Per Serving):

Calories 215, Fat9 g, Carbohydrates 10g, Fiber 3g, Protein 24g

Berry Chops Dinner

Recipe Time: 25 minutes

Serving Size: 4

Meal Type: Dinner

Diet Type: Gluten Free, Dairy Free, Soy Free, Nut Free

Ingredients:

- 2 pounds pork chops
- ½ teaspoon thyme, dried
- 2 tablespoons water
- 1 teaspoon cinnamon powder
- (ground) black pepper and salt to taste
- 12 ounces blackberries
- ½ cup balsamic vinegar

Cooking Instructions:

1. Season pork chops with salt, pepper, cinnamon and thyme.
2. Heat up a cooking pot; add the blackberries and heat over medium heat.
3. Add the vinegar, water, salt and pepper, stir the mix.
4. Simmer for 3-5 minutes and take it off the heat.
5. Brush the pork chops with half of the blueberry mix.

6. Preheat your grill and grill the chops over medium heat for 6 minutes on each side.

7. Divide the pork chops between serving plates; top with the rest of the blackberry sauce. Serve warm.

Nutritional Values (Per Serving):

Calories 286, Fat 6g, Carbohydrates 11g, Fiber 6g, Protein 22g

Cauliflower Lamb Meal

Recipe Time: 25 minutes

Serving Size: 4

Meal Type: Dinner

Diet Type: Gluten Free, Soy Free, Nut Free

Ingredients:

Mash:

- 1 large head cauliflower, cut into florets
- ½ teaspoon garlic powder
- ½ teaspoon salt
- Dash cayenne pepper

Lamb:

- 2 (8-ounce) grass-fed lamb fillets
- 2 tablespoons avocado oil
- 1 teaspoon dried rosemary
- 1 teaspoon salt
- ½ teaspoon freshly ground black pepper

Cooking Instructions:

1. In a cooking (you can also use a saucepan); add the cauliflower and water to cover it.

2. Heat it over medium stove flame. Boil and cook for 10 minutes. Drain water and transfer the cauliflower to a food processor (or blender).

3. Add the ghee, garlic powder, salt, and cayenne pepper. Blend to a smooth consistency.

4. Season the lamb with the salt and pepper.

5. In a skillet (you can also use a saucepan); heat the oil over medium stove flame.

6. Add the lamb, rosemary and cook, while stirring, until becomes evenly brown for 8-10 minutes.

7. Slice the lamb into coins and serve with the cauliflower mash.

Nutritional Values (Per Serving):

Calories 294, Fat 17g, Carbohydrates 11g, Fiber 3g, Protein 36g

Grilled Mint Chops

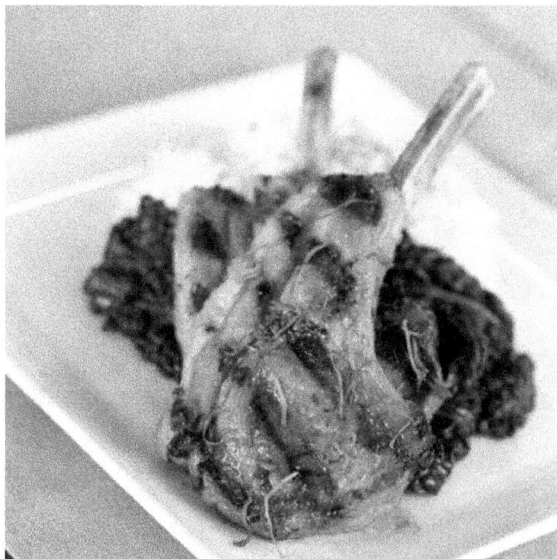

Recipe Time: 20 minutes

Serving Size: 4

Meal Type: Dinner

Diet Type: Gluten Free, Dairy Free, Soy Free, Nut Free

Ingredients:

- 8 lamb chops
- ¼ cup white vinegar
- ½ cup olive oil
- 1 cup mint leaves

- ¼ cup parsley leaves

- 2 garlic cloves, minced

- (ground) black pepper and salt to the taste

- ¼ teaspoon red pepper flakes

Cooking Instructions:

1. In a blender, add the mint, parsley, vinegar, oil, garlic, salt, pepper and pepper flakes, blend to make a smooth mix.

2. Coat the pork chops with this mix and marinate for 30-60 minutes.

3. Place the chops on the preheated grill; cook over medium-high heat for 6-7 minutes on each side.

4. Add in serving plates and serve with the leftover the mint sauce.

Nutritional Values (Per Serving):

Calories 256, Fat 8g, Carbohydrates 9g, Fiber 1g, Protein 24g

Sprouts Pork Chops

Recipe Time: 30 minutes

Serving Size: 4

Meal Type: Dinner

Diet Type: Gluten Free, Dairy Free, Soy Free, Nut Free

Ingredients:

- 1 pound pork chops, boneless

- 1 teaspoon mustard

- ½ tablespoon balsamic vinegar

- ¼ cup onion, chopped

- A pinch of (ground) black pepper and salt

- 1 ½ tablespoons olive oil

- 1 ¼ cup Brussels sprouts, halved

- 2/3 cup chicken stock

- ¼ cup applesauce, unsweetened

- 2 garlic cloves, minced

- 1 tablespoon rosemary, chopped

- 1 tablespoon sage, chopped

Cooking Instructions:

1. In a skillet (you can also use a saucepan); heat half the oil over medium stove flame.

2. Add the chops, salt, pepper, and cook, while stirring, until becomes evenly brown.

3. Transfer to a plate.

4. In the pan, heat rest of the oil, add the stock, mustard, vinegar, onion, applesauce, garlic, rosemary and sage.

5. Stir well and simmer the mix; cook for 5-6 minutes.

6. Add the sprouts, toss and cook for 4-5 minutes.

7. Add the pork chops, toss, cook mixture for a 2-3 minutes. Add in serving plates and serve.

Nutritional Values (Per Serving):

Calories 254, Fat 6g, Carbohydrates 11g, Fiber 7g, Protein 19g

Fish & Seafood

Shrimp Mushroom Squash

Recipe Time: 20 minutes

Serving Size: 4

Meal Type: Lunch

Diet Type: Gluten Free, Dairy Free, Soy Free, Nut Free

Ingredients:

- 2 tablespoons hemp seeds
- 2 tablespoons olive oil
- 1 pound shrimp, peeled and deveined
- ¼ cup coconut aminos
- 2 tablespoons raw honey
- 2 teaspoons sesame oil
- 1 yellow onion, chopped
- 4 ounces shiitake mushrooms, (cut into slices)
- 2 garlic cloves, minced
- 1 red bell pepper, (cut into slices)
- 1 yellow squash, peeled and cubed
- 2 cups chard, chopped

Cooking Instructions:

1. In a bowl (medium size), mix the aminos, honey, sesame oil and hemp seeds.

2. In a skillet (you can also use a saucepan); heat the oil over medium stove flame.

3. Add the onions, stir the mixture and cook while stirring for about 2-3 minutes until softened.

4. Add the bell pepper, squash, mushrooms and garlic, stir-cook for 5 minutes.

5. Add the shrimp and aminos mix; stir-cook for 4 minutes more.

6. Add the chard, toss; add into serving bowls and serve.

Nutritional Values (Per Serving):

Calories 236, Fat 8g, Carbohydrates 11g, Fiber 5g, Protein 9g

Spinach Sea Bass Lunch

Recipe Time: 30 minutes

Serving Size: 2

Meal Type: Lunch

Diet Type: Gluten Free, Dairy Free, Soy Free, Nut Free

Ingredients:

- 2 sea bass fillets, boneless
- 2 shallots, chopped
- Juice of ½ lemon
- 1 garlic clove, minced
- 5 cherry tomatoes, halved
- 1 tablespoon parsley, chopped
- 1 tablespoon olive oil
- 8 ounces baby spinach

Cooking Instructions:

1. Preheat an oven to 450°F. Grease a baking dish with some cooking spray.
2. Add the fish, tomatoes, parsley and garlic, drizzle the lemon juice.
3. Cover the dish and bake for 12-15 minutes and add in serving plates.

4. In a skillet (you can also use a saucepan); heat the oil over medium stove flame.

5. Add the shallots, stir the mixture and cook while stirring for about 1-2 minutes until softened.

6. Add the spinach, stir, cook for 4-5 minutes more. Add with the fish and serve warm.

Nutritional Values (Per Serving):

Calories 218, Fat 3g, Carbohydrates 11g, Fiber 6g, Protein 24g

Garlic Cod Meal

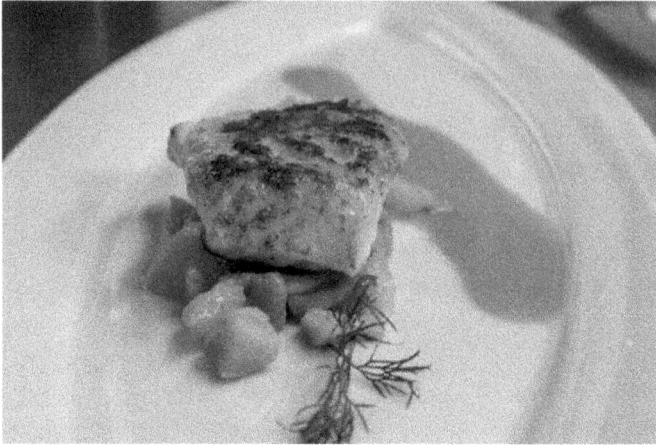

Recipe Time: 35 minutes

Serving Size: 4

Meal Type: Lunch

Diet Type: Gluten Free, Dairy Free, Soy Free, Nut Free

Ingredients:

- 2 tablespoons olive oil
- 2 tablespoons tarragon, chopped
- ¼ cup parsley, chopped
- 4 cod fillets, skinless
- 3 garlic cloves, minced
- 1 yellow onion, chopped

- (ground) black pepper and salt to the taste

- Juice of 1 lemon

- 1 lemon, (cut into slices)

- 1 tablespoon thyme, chopped

- 4 cups water

Cooking Instructions:

1. In a skillet (you can also use a saucepan); heat the oil over medium stove flame.

2. Add the onions, garlic, stir the mixture and cook while stirring for about 2-3 minutes until softened.

3. Add the salt, pepper, tarragon, parsley, thyme, water, lemon juice and lemon slices.

4. Boil the mix; add the cod, cook for 12-15 minutes, drain the liquid.

5. Serve with a side salad.

Nutritional Values (Per Serving):

Calories 181, Fat 3g, Carbohydrates 9g, Fiber 4g, Protein 12g

Cod Cucumber Delight

Recipe Time: 25 minutes

Serving Size: 4

Meal Type: Lunch

Diet Type: Gluten Free, Dairy Free, Soy Free, Nut Free

Ingredients:

- 1 tablespoon capers, drained

- 4 tablespoons + 1 teaspoon olive oil

- 4 cod fillets, skinless and boneless

- 2 tablespoons mustard

- 1 tablespoon tarragon, chopped

- (ground) black pepper and salt to the taste

- 2 cups lettuce leaves, torn

- 1 small red onion, (cut into slices)

- 1 small cucumber, (cut into slices)

- 2 tablespoons lemon juice

- 2 tablespoons water

Cooking Instructions:

1. In a bowl (medium size), mix the mustard with 2 tablespoons olive oil, tarragon, capers and water, whisk well and set aside.

2. In a skillet (you can also use a saucepan); heat 1 teaspoon oil over medium stove flame.

3. Add the fish, pepper, salt and cook, while stirring, until cooks well and turn softened on both sides.

4. In a bowl (medium size), mix the cucumber, onion, lettuce, lemon juice, 2 tablespoons olive oil, salt and pepper.

5. Arrange the cod in serving plates, top with the tarragon sauce.

6. Serve with the cucumber salad.

Nutritional Values (Per Serving):

Calories 284, Fat 8g, Carbohydrates 9g, Fiber 1g, Protein 14g

Salmon Greens

Recipe Time: 30 minutes

Serving Size: 6

Meal Type: Lunch

Diet Type: Gluten Free, Dairy Free, Soy Free, Nut Free

Ingredients:

- 4 salmon fillets, boneless and skin-on
- 15 ounces Brussels sprouts, halved
- 15 ounces baby potatoes, halved
- 1 bunch asparagus, halved and trimmed
- 1 small red onion, cubed
- 3 tablespoons balsamic vinegar
- 1 tablespoon mustard
- 2 tablespoons olive oil
- 1 cup cherry tomatoes, halved
- 1 garlic clove, minced
- 1 teaspoon thyme, chopped
- A pinch of (ground) black pepper and salt

Cooking Instructions:

1. Preheat an oven to 450°F. Grease a baking dish with some cooking spray.

2. Spread the potatoes on the sheet.

3. Add the asparagus, sprouts, onion, tomatoes, vinegar, garlic, salt, pepper, thyme and oil, toss the mix.

4. Bake for 8-10 minutes.

5. Add the salmon, season with salt and pepper, bake for 10 minutes more,

6. Add the mix in serving plates and serve.

Nutritional Values (Per Serving):

Calories 253, Fat 10g, Carbohydrates 13g, Fiber 6g, Protein 9g

Oregano Lettuce Shrimp

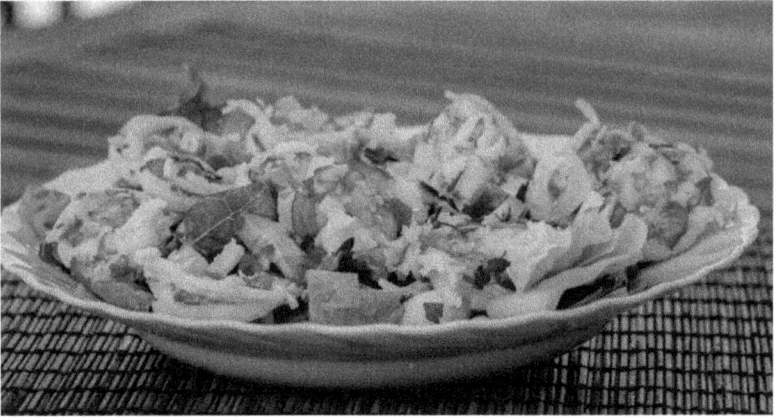

Recipe Time: 25 minutes

Serving Size: 4

Meal Type: Lunch

Diet Type: Gluten Free, Dairy Free, Soy Free, Nut Free

Ingredients:

- 3 tablespoons dill, chopped
- 1 tablespoon oregano, chopped
- 2 garlic cloves, chopped
- 1 pound shrimp, deveined and peeled
- 2 teaspoons olive oil
- 6 tablespoons lemon juice
- (ground) black pepper and salt to taste

- 2 cucumbers, (cut into slices)

- 1 red onion, (cut into slices)

- ¾ cup coconut cream

- ½ pounds cherry tomatoes

- 8 lettuce leaves

Cooking Instructions:

1. In a bowl (medium size), combine the shrimp, 1 tablespoon oregano, 2 tablespoons lemon juice, 1 tablespoon dill, and 1 teaspoon oil. Set aside for 10 minutes.

2. In another bowl, mix 1 tablespoon dill, half of the garlic, ¼ cup coconut cream, 2 tablespoons lemon juice, cucumber, salt and pepper. Combine well.

3. In another bowl, mix rest of the lemon juice, ½ cup cream, the rest of the garlic and the rest of the dill.

4. In a bowl (medium size), mix the tomatoes with onion and 1 teaspoon olive oil.

5. Heat a grill over medium-high heat, grill tomato mix and shrimp mix for 5 minutes,

6. Add them in serving plates, add the cucumber salad, lettuce leaves and other ingredients on top.

Nutritional Values (Per Serving):

Calories 268, Fat 5g, Carbohydrates 12g, Fiber 6g, Protein 11g

Mexican Pepper Salmon

Recipe Time: 25 minutes

Serving Size: 4

Meal Type: Lunch

Diet Type: Gluten Free, Dairy Free, Soy Free, Nut Free

Ingredients:

- 1 garlic clove, minced
- 1 teaspoon sweet paprika
- 4 medium salmon fillets, boneless
- 2 teaspoons olive oil
- 4 teaspoons lemon juice
- A pinch of (ground) black pepper and salt

For the salsa:

- 4 teaspoons oregano, chopped
- 1 small habanero pepper, chopped
- ¼ cup green onions, chopped
- 1 cup red bell pepper, chopped
- 1 garlic clove, minced
- ¼ cup lemon juice

Cooking Instructions:

1. In a bowl (medium size), combine the green onion, ¼ cup lemon juice, bell pepper, habanero, 1 garlic clove, oregano, black pepper and salt.

2. In a another bowl, mix the paprika, 4 teaspoons lemon juice, olive oil, and 1 garlic clove.

3. Stir the mix, cot the fish with this mix; set aside for 10 minutes.

4. Add the fish on the preheated grill over medium-high heat setting.

5. Season the fish with black pepper and salt, cook for 5 minutes on each side.

6. Add between serving plates, top with the salsa and serve.

Nutritional Values (Per Serving):

Calories 198, Fat 4g, Carbohydrates 14g, Fiber 2g, Protein 8g

Fish Curry Dinner

Recipe Time: 30 minutes

Serving Size: 4

Meal Type: Dinner

Diet Type: Gluten Free, Dairy Free, Soy Free, Nut Free

Ingredients:

- 1 tablespoon red curry paste
- 1½ cups chicken broth
- 1 (14-ounce) can coconut milk
- 1 tablespoon avocado oil
- ½ cup diced white onion
- 2 garlic cloves, minced
- ½ teaspoon coconut sugar
- 1 teaspoon salt
- ½ teaspoon ground black pepper
- 4 (4-ounce) halibut fillets

Cooking Instructions:

1. In a skillet (you can also use a saucepan); heat the oil over medium stove flame.

2. Add the onions, garlic, stir the mixture and cook while stirring for about 2-3 minutes until softened.

3. Stir in the paste. Add the broth, coconut milk, coconut sugar, salt, and pepper; combine well.

4. Reduce the heat to low and simmer for 8-10 minutes.

5. Add the fillets; cover and cook for 8-10 minutes, until flakes easily.

6. Serve the fillets with the curried broth.

Nutritional Values (Per Serving):

Calories 326, Fat 21g, Carbohydrates 13g, Fiber 2g, Protein 27g

Salmon Broccoli Bowl

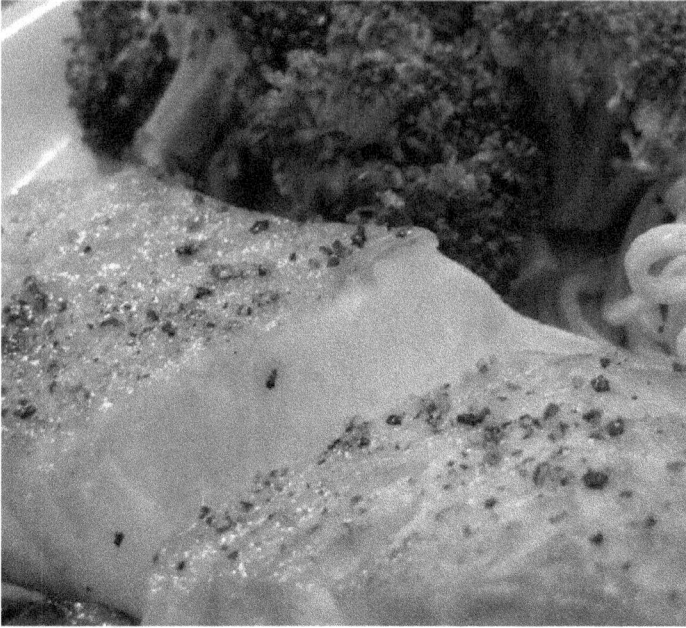

Recipe Time: 20 minutes

Serving Size: 4

Meal Type: Lunch

Diet Type: Gluten Free, Dairy Free, Soy Free, Nut Free

Ingredients:

- 3 tablespoons avocado oil

- 2 garlic cloves, minced

- 1 broccoli head, separate florets

- 1 ½ pounds salmon fillets, boneless

- A pinch of (ground) black pepper and salt

- Juice of ½ lemon

Cooking Instructions:

1. Preheat an oven to 450°F. Line a baking sheet with a foil.

2. Spread the broccoli; add the salmon, oil, garlic, salt, pepper and the lemon juice, toss gently.

3. Bake for 15 minutes.

4. Divide in serving plates and serve warm.

Nutritional Values (Per Serving):

Calories 207, Fat 6g, Carbohydrates 14g, Fiber 6g, Protein 9g

Fennel Baked Cod

Recipe Time: 25 minutes

Serving Size: 4

Meal Type: Dinner

Diet Type: Gluten Free, Dairy Free, Soy Free, Nut Free

Ingredients:

- 3 sun-dried tomatoes, chopped
- 1 small red onion, (cut into slices)
- ½ fennel bulb,(cut into slices)
- 2 cod fillets, boneless
- 1 garlic cloves, minced
- 1 teaspoon olive oil
- Black pepper to the taste
- 4 black olives, pitted and sliced
- 2 rosemary springs
- ¼ teaspoon red pepper flakes

Cooking Instructions:

1. Preheat an oven to 400°F. Grease a baking dish with some cooking spray.

2. Add the cod, garlic, black pepper, tomatoes, onion, fennel, olives, rosemary and pepper flakes; mix gently.

3. Bake for 14-15 minutes.

4. Divide the fish mix between plates and serve.

Nutritional Values (Per Serving):

Calories 255, Fat 4g, Carbohydrates 11g, Fiber 6g, Protein 16g

Beet Haddock Dinner

Recipe Time: 40-45 minutes

Serving Size: 4

Meal Type: Dinner

Diet Type: Gluten Free, Dairy Free, Soy Free, Nut Free

Ingredients:

- 2 tablespoons olive oil
- 2 tablespoons apple cider vinegar
- 1 teaspoon chopped fresh thyme
- 8 beets, peeled and cut into small chunks
- 2 shallots, (cut into slices)
- 1 teaspoon minced garlic
- Pinch sea salt to taste
- 4 (5-ounce) haddock fillets, patted dry

Cooking Instructions:

1. Preheat an oven to 400°F. Grease a baking dish with some cooking spray.
2. In a bowl (medium size), mix the beets, shallots, garlic, and 1 tablespoon olive oil.
3. Add the beet mixture in the baking dish.
4. Bake for about 25-30 minutes, or until the vegetables are caramelized.

5. Remove from oven and stir in the cider vinegar, thyme, and sea salt.

6. In a skillet (you can also use a saucepan); heat the remaining oil over medium stove flame.

7. Add the fish, stir the mixture and cook while stirring for 12-15 minutes until cooks well.

8. Flake the fish and serve with roasted beets.

Nutritional Values (Per Serving):

Calories 324, Fat 8g, Carbohydrates 22g, Fiber 3g, Protein 37g

Honey Scallops

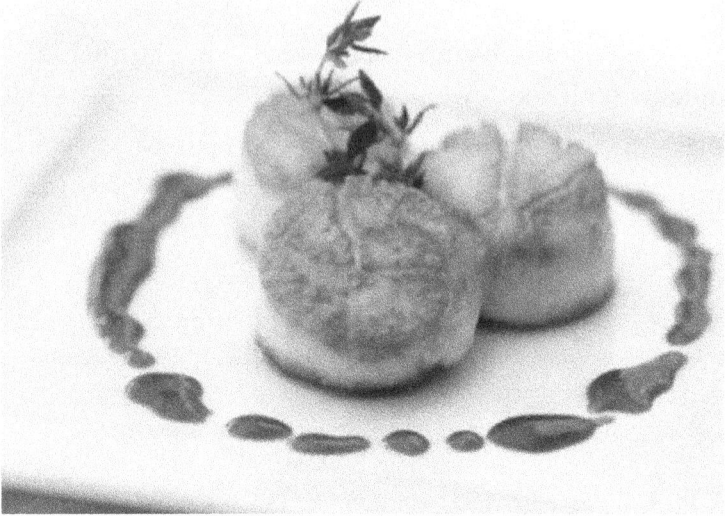

Recipe Time: 25 minutes

Serving Size: 4

Meal Type: Dinner

Diet Type: Gluten Free, Dairy Free, Soy Free, Nut Free

Ingredients:

- 1 pound large scallops, rinsed

- Dash of ground black pepper and salt to taste

- 3 tablespoons coconut aminos

- 2 garlic cloves, minced

- 2 tablespoons avocado oil

- ¼ cup raw honey

- 1 tablespoon apple cider vinegar

Cooking Instructions:

1. Sprinkle the scallops with the salt and pepper.

2. In a skillet (you can also use a saucepan); heat the oil over medium stove flame.

3. Add the scallops, stir the mixture and cook while stirring for about 2-3 minutes until softened and golden.

4. Transfer to a plate, and set aside.

5. In the same skillet or pan, heat the honey, coconut aminos, garlic, and vinegar.

6. Cook for 6-7 minutes; add the scallops and coat well. Serve warm.

Nutritional Values (Per Serving):

Calories 346, Fat 17g, Carbohydrates 27g, Fiber 2g, Protein 21g

Kale Cod Secret

Recipe Time: 30 minutes

Serving Size: 4

Meal Type: Dinner

Diet Type: Gluten Free, Dairy Free, Soy Free, Nut Free

Ingredients:

- 4 cod fillets, skinless and boneless
- 1 tablespoon ginger, (shredded or grated)
- 4 teaspoons lemon zest
- A pinch of (ground) black pepper and salt
- 3 leeks, chopped
- 2 cups veggie stock
- 2 tablespoons lemon juice
- 2 tablespoons olive oil
- 1 pound kale, chopped
- ½ teaspoon sesame oil

Cooking Instructions:

1. In a bowl (medium size), mix the zest with salt and pepper. Coat the fish with this mix.

2. In a skillet (you can also use a saucepan); heat the leeks, ginger and lemon juice over medium stove flame.

3. Heat for a few minutes; add the fish fillets.

4. Cover and cook for 8-10 minutes, transfer it to a plate.

5. Strain the liquid and reserve the leeks. Add the fish in serving plates.

6. In a skillet (you can also use a saucepan); heat the oil over medium stove flame.

7. Add the kale, stir the mixture and cook while stirring for about 3-4 minutes until softened.

8. Add the soup liquid and cook for 4-5 minutes more.

9. Add the reserved leeks; cook for 2 minutes.

10. Divide into fish bowls, drizzle the sesame oil all over and serve.

Nutritional Values (Per Serving):

Calories 238, Fat 3g, Carbohydrates 12g, Fiber 4g, Protein 16g

Scrumptious Coconut Shrimps

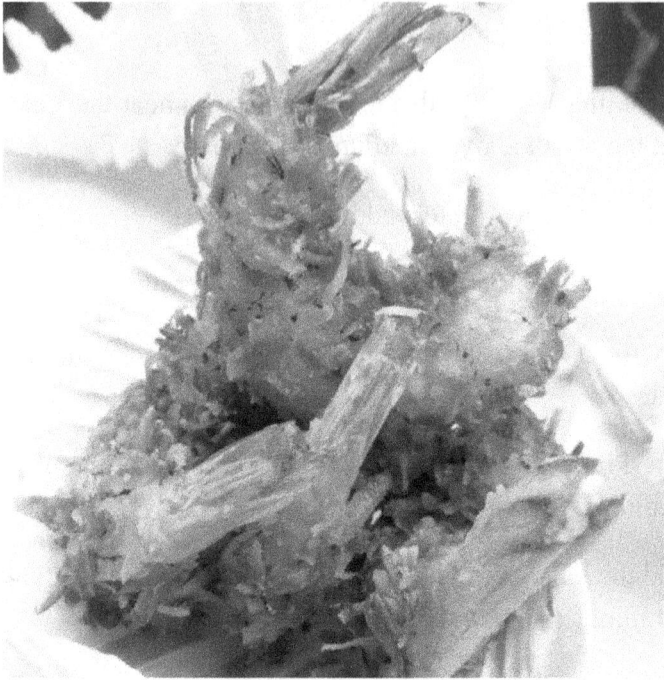

Recipe Time: 15-20 minutes

Serving Size: 4

Meal Type: Dinner

Diet Type: Gluten Free, Dairy Free, Soy Free, Nut Free

Ingredients:

- 2 eggs

- 1 cup dried shredded coconut, unsweetened

- ¼ teaspoon paprika

- Dash cayenne pepper

- ¼ cup coconut flour

- ½ teaspoon salt

- Dash freshly ground black pepper

- ¼ cup coconut oil

- 1 pound raw shrimp, peeled and deveined

Cooking Instructions:

1. In a bowl, whisk the eggs.

2. In another bowl, mix the coconut, flour, salt, paprika, cayenne pepper, and black pepper.

3. Coat the shrimp into the egg mixture, and then into the coconut mix.

4. In a skillet (you can also use a saucepan); heat the oil over medium stove flame.

5. Add the shrimps and cook for 2-3 minutes per side. Serve warm.

Nutritional Values (Per Serving):

Calories 246, Fat 18g, Carbohydrates 8g, Fiber 3g, Protein 19g

Herbed Mussels Treat

Recipe Time: 30 minutes

Serving Size: 4

Meal Type: Dinner

Diet Type: Gluten Free, Dairy Free, Soy Free, Nut Free

Ingredients:

- 1 tablespoon olive oil
- 2 teaspoons minced garlic
- 1 cup coconut milk
- ½ cup chicken bone broth
- 2 teaspoons chopped fresh thyme
- 1 teaspoon chopped fresh oregano
- 1½ pounds mussels, scrubbed and debearded
- 1 scallion, sliced white and green parts

Cooking Instructions:

1. In a skillet (you can also use a saucepan); heat the oil over medium stove flame.

2. Add the garlic, stir the mixture and cook while stirring for about 2-3 minutes until softened.

3. Add the coconut milk, broth, thyme, and oregano.

4. Boil the mix and add the mussels. Cover and cook for about 8 minutes, or until the shells opened up.

5. Remove any unopened shells and add in the scallion; serve warm.

Nutritional Values (Per Serving):

Calories 318, Fat 21g, Carbohydrates 12g, Fiber 2g, Protein 23g

Coconut Chili Salmon

Recipe Time: 25 minutes

Serving Size: 6

Meal Type: Dinner

Diet Type: Gluten Free, Dairy Free, Soy Free, Nut Free

Ingredients:

- 1 ¼ cups coconut, shredded
- 2 tablespoons olive oil
- ¼ cup water
- 1 pound salmon, cubed
- 1/3 cup coconut flour
- A pinch of (ground) black pepper and salt
- 1 egg
- 4 red chilies, chopped
- 3 garlic cloves, minced
- ¼ cup balsamic vinegar
- ½ cup raw honey

Cooking Instructions:

1. In a bowl (medium size), mix the flour with a pinch of salt.

2. In another bowl, whisk the egg and black pepper.

3. Add the shredded coconut in another bowl.

4. Coat the salmon cubes in flour, egg and coconut mix one by one.

5. In a skillet (you can also use a saucepan); heat the oil over medium stove flame.

6. Add the salmon, stir-fry them for 2-3 minutes on each side. Place in serving plates.

7. Heat water over medium-high heat in the pan, add the chilies, cloves, vinegar and honey, stir gently.

8. Boil the mix and simmer for 4 minutes; top over the salmon and serve.

Nutritional Values (Per Serving):

Calories 218, Fat 5g, Carbohydrates 14g, Fiber 2g, Protein 17g

Vegan & Vegetarian

Cauliflower Coconut Curry

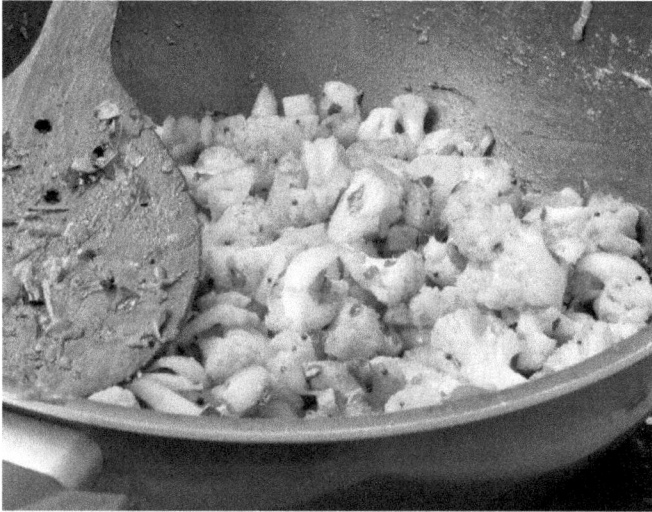

Recipe Time: 55 minutes

Serving Size: 4

Meal Type: Lunch

Diet Type: Gluten Free, Dairy Free, Soy Free, Nut Free, Vegan, Vegetarian

Ingredients:

- 3 cups vegetable stock

- 3 pounds cauliflower, florets separated

- 2 garlic cloves, minced

- 2 carrots, chopped

- 1 yellow onion, chopped

- 1 tablespoon coconut oil

- A pinch of (ground) black pepper and salt

- ½ cup coconut milk

- A pinch of nutmeg

- A pinch of cayenne pepper

- A handful parsley, chopped

Cooking Instructions:

1. In a skillet (you can also use a saucepan); heat the oil over medium stove flame.

2. Add the onions, carrots, garlic, stir the mixture and cook while stirring for about 4-5 minutes until softened.

3. Add the cauliflower and stock. Boil the mix and reduce heat; cover, cook for 40-45 minutes.

4. Add the mix to a blender, add the milk, salt and pepper.

5. Blend well and add into the bowls; sprinkle nutmeg, cayenne and parsley. Serve warm.

Nutritional Values (Per Serving):

Calories 234, Fat 2g, Carbohydrates 11g, Fiber 5g, Protein 7g

Pomegranate Kale Salad

Recipe Time: 15 minutes

Serving Size: 4

Meal Type: Lunch

Diet Type: Gluten Free, Dairy Free, Soy Free, Nut Free, Vegan, Vegetarian

Ingredients:

- ¼ cup shelled sunflower seeds
- 2 tablespoons lemon juice
- 2 bunches kale, stemmed and chopped
- 3 scallions, (cut into slices)
- 1 avocado, diced
- 3 tablespoons extra-virgin olive oil
- ½ teaspoon salt
- Freshly ground black pepper
- ¼ cup pomegranate pips

Cooking Instructions:

1. In a mixing bowl, combine the kale, scallions, avocado, sunflower seeds, lemon juice, olive oil, and salt, and pepper.

2. Combine well.

3. Mix the pomegranate seeds and serve fresh.

Nutritional Values (Per Serving):

Calories 243, Fat 18g, Carbohydrates 13g, Fiber 5g, Protein 6g

Black Bean Chili Potato

Recipe Time: 25 minutes

Serving Size: 7-8

Meal Type: Dinner

Diet Type: Gluten Free, Dairy Free, Soy Free, Nut Free, Vegan, Vegetarian

Ingredients:

- 1 red bell pepper, diced
- 1 green bell pepper, diced
- 3 cups cooked sweet potato cubes
- 2 tablespoons avocado oil
- 1 red onion, diced
- 5 garlic cloves, minced
- 1 (28-ounce) can diced tomatoes with their juice
- 1 tablespoon lime juice
- 3 cups cooked black beans, drained and rinsed well
- 2 cups vegetable broth
- 1 teaspoon ground cumin
- 1 teaspoon salt

- 1 tablespoon chili powder

- 1 teaspoon cocoa powder

- ½ teaspoon ground cinnamon

- ¼ teaspoon cayenne pepper

- ¼ teaspoon dried oregano

Cooking Instructions:

1. In a cooking pot (you can also use a deep saucepan); heat the oil over medium stove flame.

2. Add the onions, garlic, stir the mixture and cook while stirring for about 2-3 minutes until softened.

3. Add the red bell pepper and green bell pepper; stir-cook for about 3 minutes until soft.

4. Add the other ingredients and stir to combine.

5. Bring to a simmer, and cook for 15 minutes. Serve immediately.

Nutritional Values (Per Serving):

Calories 162, Fat 4g, Carbohydrates 28g, Fiber 6g, Protein 8g

Chickpea Veggie Lunch

Recipe Time: 35 minutes

Serving Size: 4

Meal Type: Lunch

Diet Type: Gluten Free, Dairy Free, Soy Free, Nut Free, Vegan, Vegetarian

Ingredients:

- 1 teaspoon sweet paprika

- 2 teaspoons turmeric powder

- 1 tablespoon coconut oil

- 15 ounces canned chickpeas, drained

- 8 small potatoes, cubed

- ¼ cup quinoa

- A pinch of (ground) black pepper and salt

- ½ tablespoon olive oil

- 2 kale leaves, chopped

- 1 avocado, pitted, peeled and sliced

Cooking Instructions:

1. Preheat an oven to 450°F. Line two baking sheets with a foil.

2. Place the potatoes on the sheet, drizzle the coconut oil over.

3. Sprinkle 1 teaspoon turmeric, and season with salt and pepper.

4. Bake for 5 minutes and set aside.

5. In a bowl (medium size), mix the chickpeas with the paprika, toss.

6. Place them over another baking sheet. Bake for 20 minutes at 350°F.

7. In a mixing bowl, mix the potatoes with the chickpeas.

8. Add the rest of the turmeric, olive oil, salt, pepper, quinoa, kale and avocado.

9. Toss and serve.

Nutritional Values (Per Serving):

Calories 291, Fat 4g, Carbohydrates 15g, Fiber 6g, Protein 8g

Fruit Blast Salad

Recipe Time: 15 minutes

Serving Size: 6

Meal Type: Lunch

Diet Type: Gluten Free, Dairy Free, Soy Free, Vegetarian

Ingredients:

- 1 cup nectarines, sliced
- ½ cup pecans, chopped
- ¼ cup red onion, thinly sliced
- 4 cups mixed chopped greens
- 1 cup peaches, sliced
- 1 cup cherries, pitted and halved
- ¼ cup basil leaves
- 1 tablespoon lemon juice
- ½ tablespoon raw honey
- ⅓ cup extra-virgin olive oil
- ¼ cup balsamic vinegar
- Dash salt and ground black pepper to taste

Cooking Instructions:

1. In a mixing bowl, combine the greens, peaches, cherries, nectarines, pecans, red onion, and basil.

2. In another bowl, add the olive oil, vinegar, lemon juice, honey, salt and pepper. Combine well.

3. Pour the dressing mix over the salad. Toss well and serve.

Nutritional Values (Per Serving):

Calories 219, Fat 18g, Carbohydrates 17g, Fiber 3g, Protein 2g

Avocado Quinoa Salad

Recipe Time: 5 minutes

Serving Size: 2

Meal Type: Lunch

Diet Type: Gluten Free, Dairy Free, Soy Free, Vegan, Vegetarian

Ingredients:

- 1 medium bunch collard greens, chopped

- 4 tablespoons walnuts, chopped

- 1 cup quinoa, cooked

- 1 avocado, chopped

- 2 tablespoons white wine vinegar

- 1 tablespoon olive oil

- 1 tablespoon maple syrup

Cooking Instructions:

1. In a bowl (medium size), combine the quinoa, avocado, greens, walnuts, vinegar, oil and maple syrup.

2. Toss well and serve.

Nutritional Values (Per Serving):

Calories 168, Fat 3g, Carbohydrates 6g, Fiber 2g, Protein 3g

Chickpea Patties

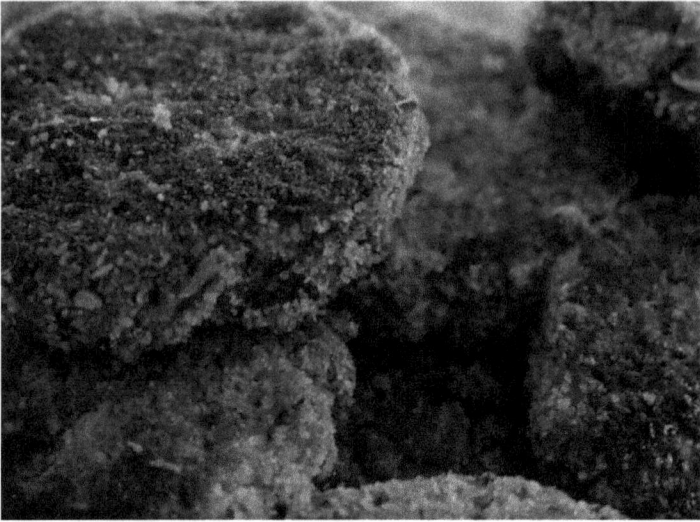

Recipe Time: 20 minutes

Serving Size: 4

Meal Type: Lunch

Diet Type: Gluten Free, Dairy Free, Soy Free, Nut Free, Vegan, Vegetarian

Ingredients:

- ¼ cup parsley leaves

- 2 tablespoons coconut flour

- 2 tablespoons chickpeas flour

- 2 garlic cloves, peeled

- 1 yellow onion, peeled and chopped

- 1 ½ cups canned chickpeas, drained and rinsed

- 1 teaspoon turmeric powder

- A pinch of (ground) black pepper and salt

- A pinch of cayenne pepper

- 3 tablespoons coconut or olive oil

Cooking Instructions:

1. In a blender, mix the garlic with the onion, chickpeas, parsley, coconut flour, turmeric, salt, pepper and cayenne.

2. Make patties from the mix. Coat them in the chickpeas flour.

3. In a skillet (you can also use a saucepan); heat the oil over medium stove flame.

4. Cook the patties for 4-5 minutes on each side.

5. Serve with your choice of dip or fresh chopped veggies.

Nutritional Values (Per Serving):

Calories 249, Fat 4g, Carbohydrates 14g, Fiber 4g, Protein 8g

Chickpea Raisin Curry

Recipe Time: 20 minutes

Serving Size: 4

Meal Type: Dinner

Diet Type: Gluten Free, Soy Free, Vegetarian

Ingredients:

- 1 red bell pepper, chopped

- 1 ½ cups vegetable broth

- 1 tablespoon curry powder

- 2 small white onions, diced

- 2 garlic cloves, minced

- 2 tablespoons avocado oil

- ½ teaspoon salt

- 2 cups cooked chickpeas, rinsed and drained

- ½ cup golden raisins

- 1 medium apple, diced

- ½ cup cashews, roughly chopped

- ½ cup plain whole-milk yogurt (optional)

Cooking Instructions:

1. In a skillet (you can also use a saucepan); heat the oil over medium stove flame.

2. Add the onions, garlic, stir the mixture and cook while stirring for about 2-3 minutes until softened.

3. Add the bell pepper, and sauté for 4-5 minutes.

4. Add the broth, curry powder, and salt; combine and bring to a simmer.

5. Add the chickpeas, apple, and raisins; cook for 4-5 minutes.

6. Mix in the cashews. Serve warm with the yogurt on top.

Nutritional Values (Per Serving):

Calories 378, Fat 17g, Carbohydrates 38g, Fiber 12g, Protein 11g

Zucchini Buckwheat Pasta

Recipe Time: 15 minutes

Serving Size: 4

Meal Type: Dinner

Diet Type: Gluten Free, Soy Free, Vegetarian

Ingredients:

Pesto:

- ¼ cup shelled sunflower seeds
- 2 garlic cloves
- 1 cup basil leaves
- 1 cup chopped zucchini
- ½ cup extra-virgin olive oil, divided
- ¼ cup raw Parmesan cheese, shredded
- 1 teaspoon lemon juice
- ¼ teaspoon salt
- Freshly ground black pepper

Pasta:

- 8 ounces buckwheat pasta

Cooking Instructions:

1. Cook the pasta in water as directed on pack.

2. In a food processor (or blender), puree the basil, zucchini, sunflower seeds, garlic, and ¼ cup of olive oil.

3. Add the cheese, lemon juice, salt, and pepper. Blend to combine well.

4. Add the remaining oil and blend well.

5. Serve the pesto with the pasta and top with sunflower seeds.

Nutritional Values (Per Serving):

Calories 426, Fat 25g, Carbohydrates 34g, Fiber 4g, Protein 9g

Brown Rice Lentils

Recipe Time: 30 minutes

Serving Size: 4

Meal Type: Dinner

Diet Type: Gluten Free, Dairy Free, Soy Free, Nut Free, Vegan, Vegetarian

Ingredients:

- 1 celery stalk, finely chopped
- 1 carrot, minced
- 2 garlic cloves, minced
- 2 tablespoons avocado oil
- 1 small white onion, chopped
- 7 tablespoons tomato paste
- 2 tablespoons apple cider vinegar
- 1 pound cooked lentils
- ½ red bell pepper, finely chopped
- 1 tablespoon pure maple syrup
- 1 teaspoon Dijon mustard
- 1 teaspoon chili powder
- ½ teaspoon dried oregano
- Cooked brown rice or wild rice to serve

Cooking Instructions:

1. In a skillet (you can also use a saucepan); heat the oil over medium stove flame.

2. Add the onion, celery, carrot, and garlic, stir the mixture and cook while stirring for about 4-5 minutes until softened.

3. Add the bell pepper, and sauté for 2 minutes.

4. Add the tomato paste, vinegar, maple syrup, mustard, chili powder, and oregano.

5. Reduce cooking flame and stir-cook for about 8-10 minutes.

6. Serve warm with the rice.

Nutritional Values (Per Serving):

Calories 288, Fat 7g, Carbohydrates 32g, Fiber 10g, Protein 14g

Mushroom Rice Bowl

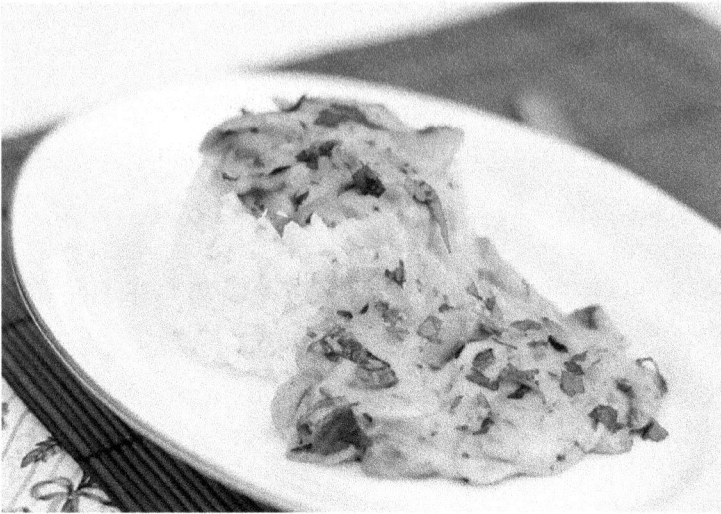

Recipe Time: 25 minutes

Serving Size: 8

Meal Type: Lunch

Diet Type: Gluten Free, Soy Free, Nut Free, Vegetarian

Ingredients:

- 1 small sweet onion, diced
- 3 garlic cloves, minced
- 2 cups cremini mushrooms, (cut into slices)
- 3 cups cooked wild rice
- 2 tablespoons ghee

- ½ cup vegetable broth

- ½ teaspoon dried thyme

- ½ teaspoon salt

Cooking Instructions:

1. Place the rice in a bowl and set aside.

2. In a skillet (you can also use a saucepan); heat the ghee over medium stove flame.

3. Add the onions, garlic, stir the mixture and cook while stirring for about 4-5 minutes until softened.

4. Stir in the mushrooms, broth, thyme, and salt; stir-cook for 8-10 minutes until the mushrooms are tender.

5. Add the mixture to the rice and serve warm.

Nutritional Values (Per Serving):

Calories 148, Fat 3g, Carbohydrates 23g, Fiber 2g, Protein 5g

Chickpea Lettuce Wraps

Recipe Time: 15 minutes

Serving Size: 2

Meal Type: Lunch or Dinner

Diet Type: Gluten Free, Dairy Free, Soy Free, Nut Free, Vegetarian

Ingredients:

- ½ shallot, minced
- 1 green apple, cored and diced
- 3 tablespoons tahini (sesame paste)
- 1 (15-ounce) can chickpeas, drained and rinsed well
- 1 celery stalk, diced
- 1 teaspoon Dijon mustard
- 2 teaspoons lemon juice
- 1 teaspoon raw honey
- Dash salt to taste
- 4 romaine lettuce leaves

Cooking Instructions:

1. In a bowl (medium size), combine the chickpeas, celery, shallot, apple, tahini, lemon juice, honey, mustard, and salt. Combine well.

2. Add the mix over the romaine lettuce leaves on a plate.

3. Wrap the leaves and serve.

Nutritional Values (Per Serving):

Calories 317, Fat 14g, Carbohydrates 31g, Fiber 12g, Protein 15g

Snacks & Sauces

Avocado Prosciutto Snack

Recipe Time: 5 minutes

Serving Size/Yield: 12

Diet Type: Gluten Free, Dairy Free, Soy Free, Nut Free

Ingredients:

- 2 large avocados, halved, pitted

- 12 slices prosciutto

- 2 apples, each cut into 6 pieces

- Raw honey (optional)

Cooking Instructions:

1. Take each avocado halves and make 3 slices from each half.

2. Take 1 prosciutto slice; place 1 avocado slice and 1 apple slice at one end and roll to make a wrap. Repeat the same.

3. Top with the honey and serve.

Nutritional Values (Per Serving):

Calories 238, Fat 17g, Carbohydrates 11g, Fiber 5g, Protein 16g

Honey Bean Dip

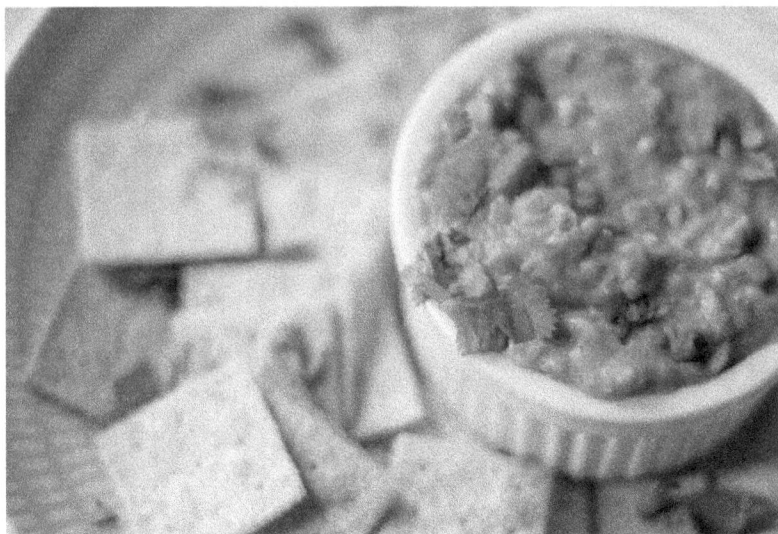

Recipe Time: 5 minutes

Serving Size/Yield: 3-4 cups

Diet Type: Gluten Free, Dairy Free, Soy Free, Nut Free, Vegetarian

Ingredients:

- 2 cherry tomatoes

- 2 tablespoons filtered water

- 1 tablespoon apple cider vinegar

- 1 (14-ounce) can each of kidney beans and black beans

- 2 garlic cloves

- ¼ teaspoon ground cumin

- ¼ teaspoon salt

- 2 teaspoons raw honey

- 1 teaspoon lime juice

- Pinch cayenne pepper to taste

- Freshly ground black pepper to taste

Cooking Instructions:

1. In a blender or food processor, add the beans, garlic, tomatoes, water, vinegar, honey, lime juice, cumin, salt, cayenne pepper, and black pepper.

2. Blend until turns smooth. Add the mix in a bowl.

3. Cover and refrigerate to chill. You can refrigerate for up to 5 days.

Nutritional Values (Per Serving ½ cup):

Calories 158, Fat 1g, Carbohydrates 33g, Fiber 8g, Protein 9g

Bean Potato Spread

Recipe Time: 25 minutes

Serving Size: 7-8

Diet Type: Gluten Free, Dairy Free, Soy Free, Nut Free, Vegan, Vegetarian

Ingredients:

- 2 tablespoons lime juice

- 1 tablespoon olive oil

- 5 garlic cloves, minced

- 1 cup canned garbanzo beans, drained and rinsed

- 4 cups cooked sweet potatoes, peeled and chopped

- ¼ cup sesame paste

- ½ teaspoon cumin, ground

- 2 tablespoons water

- A pinch of salt

Cooking Instructions:

1. In a blender, add all the ingredients and blend to make a smooth mix.

2. Transfer to a bowl.

3. Serve with carrot, celery or veggie sticks.

Nutritional Values (Per Serving):

Calories 156, Fat 3g, Carbohydrates 10g, Fiber 6g, Protein 8g

Zucchini Crisps

Recipe Time: 30 minutes

Serving Size/Yield: 12 pieces

Diet Type: Gluten Free, Soy Free, Nut Free, Vegan, Vegetarian

Ingredients:

- ½ cup almond flour
- 1 medium zucchini, peeled and halved widthwise
- 1 tablespoon avocado oil
- ½ teaspoon salt
- ½ teaspoon garlic powder
- ½ teaspoon ground black pepper

Cooking Instructions:

1. Preheat an oven to 425°F. Line a baking sheet with a foil.

2. In a mixing bowl, mix the flour, salt, garlic powder, and pepper.

3. Make total 12 strips from zucchini halves.

4. Brush the strips with the oil, and coat with the flour mixture. Evenly space the fries on the prepared sheet.

5. Bake for 20 minutes, or until crispy. Serve warm.

Nutritional Values (Per Piece):

Calories 42, Fat 3g, Carbohydrates 2g, Fiber 0.3g, Protein 1g

Evening Chicken Bites

Recipe Time: 20 minutes

Serving Size: 2

Diet Type: Gluten Free, Dairy Free, Soy Free

Ingredients:

- 2 tablespoons garlic powder

- 2 chicken breasts, cubed

- ½ cup almond flour

- 1 egg

- (ground) black pepper and salt to the taste

- ½ cup coconut oil

Cooking Instructions:

1. In a bowl (medium size), mix the garlic powder, flour, salt and pepper and stir.

2. In another bowl, whisk the egg.

3. Coat the chicken breast cubes in egg mix, then coat with the flour mix.

4. In a skillet (you can also use a saucepan); heat the oil over medium stove flame.

5. Add the chicken pieces, cook them for 4-5 minutes on each side until cooks well.

6. Serve warm.

Nutritional Values (Per Serving):

Calories 72, Fat 4g, Carbohydrates 6g, Fiber 2g, Protein 8g

Cashew Ginger Dip

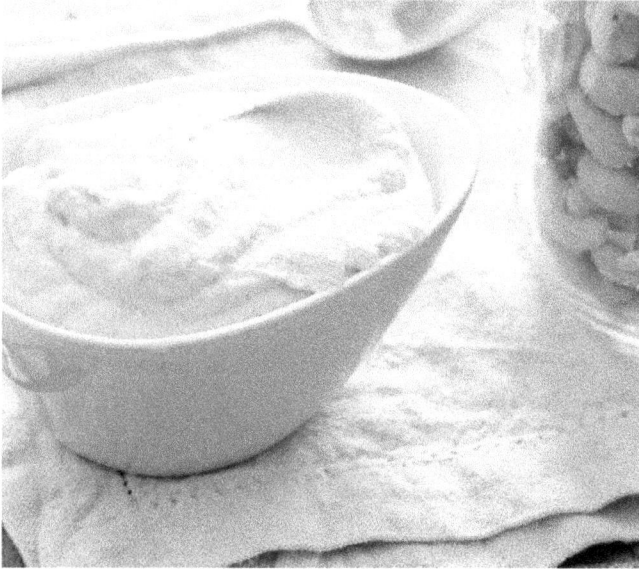

Recipe Time: 5 minutes

Serving Size/Yield: 1 cup

Diet Type: Gluten Free, Dairy Free, Soy Free, Vegan, Vegetarian

Ingredients:

- 1 tablespoon extra-virgin olive oil

- 2 teaspoons coconut aminos

- 1 cup raw cashews, soaked in filtered water for 20-25 minutes and drained

- 2 garlic cloves

- ¼ cup filtered water

- 1 teaspoon lemon juice

- ½ teaspoon ground ginger

- ¼ teaspoon salt

- Pinch cayenne pepper

Cooking Instructions:

1. In a blender or food processor, puree the cashews, garlic, water, olive oil, aminos, lemon juice, ginger, salt, and cayenne pepper.

2. Add the mix in a bowl.

3. Cover and refrigerate until chilled. You can use store it for 4-5 days in refrigerator.

Nutritional Values (Per Serving):

Calories 124, Fat 9g, Carbohydrates 5g, Fiber 1g, Protein 3g

Buckwheat Evening Delight

Recipe Time: 25 minutes

Serving Size: 4

Diet Type: Gluten Free, Dairy Free, Soy Free, Nut Free, Vegan, Vegetarian

Ingredients:

- 2 teaspoons minced garlic
- 2 cups cooked buckwheat
- 1 tablespoon olive oil
- ½ cup chopped red onion
- Juice of 1 lemon
- Zest of 1 lemon (optional)
- ½ cup chopped parsley
- ¼ cup chopped mint
- Sea salt to taste

Cooking Instructions:

1. In a skillet (you can also use a saucepan); heat the oil over medium stove flame.
2. Add the onions, garlic, stir the mixture and cook while stirring for about 2-3 minutes until softened.

3. Stir in the buckwheat, lemon juice, and lemon zest. Stir-cook for about 4-5 minutes.

4. Stir in the parsley and mint. Sauté for 1 minute.

5. Remove from the heat and season with salt. Serve warm.

Nutritional Values (Per Serving):

Calories 394, Fat 6g, Carbohydrates 38g, Fiber 9g, Protein 16g

Spiced Chickpeas

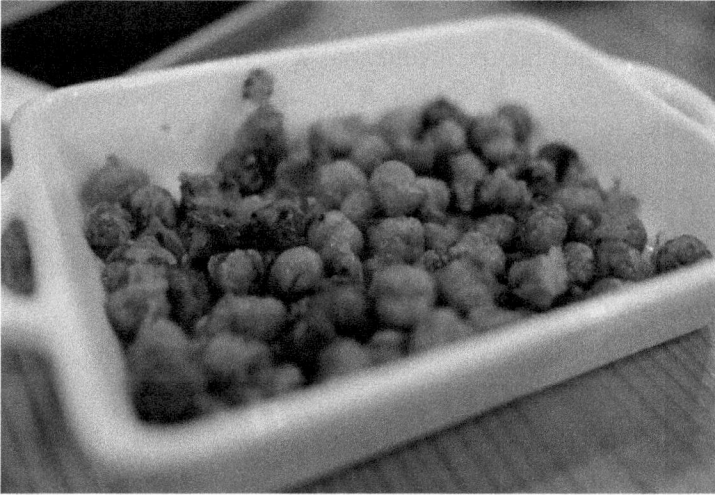

Recipe Time: 20-25 minutes

Serving Size/Yield: 4 cups

Diet Type: Gluten Free, Dairy Free, Soy Free, Nut Free, Vegan, Vegetarian

Ingredients:

- 4 cups cooked chickpeas, drained, and dried

- 1 teaspoon garlic powder

- 2 tablespoons extra-virgin olive oil

- 1 teaspoon salt

- Ground black pepper to taste

Cooking Instructions:

1. Preheat an oven to 400°F. Line a baking sheet with a foil.

2. Spread the chickpeas and coat with the oil.

3. Bake for 20 minutes, shake it in between.

4. Add them to a large bowl.

5. Toss with the salt and garlic powder; season with pepper. Serve warm.

Nutritional Values (Per Serving ¼ cup):

Calories 148, Fat 5g, Carbohydrates 22g, Fiber 6g, Protein 8g

Desserts

Blackberry Granita

Recipe Time: 10 minutes

Serving Size: 4

Diet Type: Gluten Free, Dairy Free, Soy Free, Nut Free, Vegetarian

Ingredients:

- ½ cup raw honey
- ¼ cup lemon juice
- 1 pound blackberries
- ½ cup water
- 1 teaspoon chopped thyme

Cooking Instructions:

1. In a blender or food processor, combine the blackberries, water, honey, lemon juice, and thyme.

2. Blend to make a smooth puree.

3. Process through a fine-mesh sieve into a square baking dish. D

4. Place it in the freezer for 2 hours. Remove the dish and break any frozen section by stirring gently. Free again for 1-2 hours; repeat the same until you get a granite like structure.

5. Serve chilled.

Nutritional Values (Per Serving):

Calories 176, Fat 1g, Carbohydrates 42g, Fiber 6g, Protein 2g

Spiced Fruit Blast

Recipe Time: 35 minutes

Serving Size: 4

Diet Type: Gluten Free, Dairy Free, Soy Free, Vegan, Vegetarian

Ingredients:

For Filling:

- 1 large mango, peeled and diced
- 1 pineapple, peeled and cut into small chunks
- 2 tablespoons coconut oil
- 2 tablespoons maple syrup
- 1/8 teaspoon ground cinnamon
- 1/8 teaspoon ground ginger

For Topping:

- ½ teaspoon ground allspice
- ½ teaspoon ground cinnamon
- ½ teaspoon ground ginger
- ¾ cup almonds
- 1/3 cup coconut, shredded

Cooking Instructions:

1. Preheat an oven to 375°F. Grease a baking dish with some cooking spray.

2. In a skillet (you can also use a saucepan); heat the oil over medium stove flame.

3. Add the maple syrup and cook, stirring for about 1-2 minutes.

4. Stir in remaining ingredients and cook for 4-5 minutes.

5. Remove from heat, cool down and add into a baking dish.

6. In a blender, add the topping ingredients.

7. Blend to make a meal like mixture.

8. Bake for about 15 minutes or turns golden brown. Serve warm.

Nutritional Values (Per Serving):

Calories 307, Fat 22g, Carbohydrates 26g, Fiber 4g, Protein 3g

Cherry Cobbler

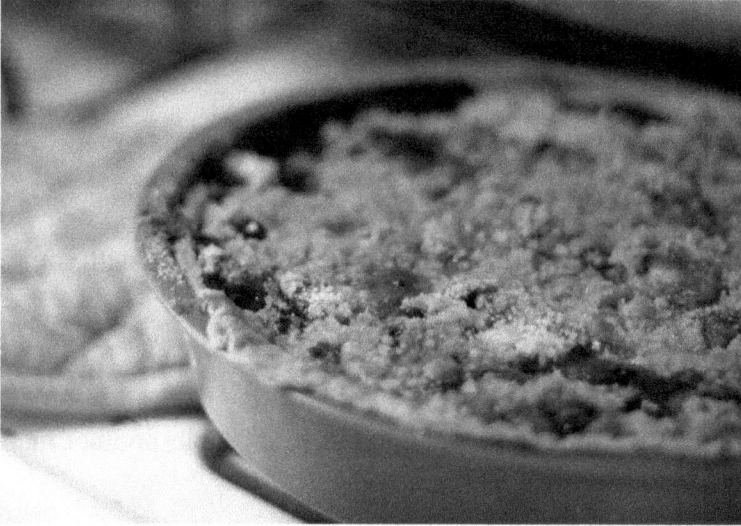

Recipe Time: 30-35 minutes

Serving Size: 4

Diet Type: Gluten Free, Dairy Free, Soy Free, Nut Free, Vegan, Vegetarian

Ingredients:

- ¼ cup unsweetened coconut, shredded

- ¼ cup coconut flour

- 1 tablespoon arrowroot flour

- 2 cups cherries, pitted

- ¼ cup +1 tablespoon cup maple syrup

- ¼ cup pecans, chopped

- ½ teaspoon ground cinnamon

- Pinch of salt

Cooking Instructions:

1. Preheat an oven to 375°F. Grease a baking dish with some cooking spray.

2. Add the cherries and ¼ cup syrup.

3. In a bowl (medium size), combine the 1 tablespoon of maple syrup and remaining ingredients.

4. Add the mixture over cherries evenly.

5. Bake for 25 minutes and serve warm.

Nutritional Values (Per Serving):

Calories 168, Fat 13g, Carbohydrates 22g, Fiber 1g, Protein 5g

Lemon Coconut Mousse

Recipe Time: 15-20 minutes

Serving Size: 4

Diet Type: Gluten Free, Dairy Free, Soy Free, Nut Free, Vegetarian

Ingredients:

- 2 cups coconut milk

- ½ cup lemon juice

- ¼ cup water

- 2 teaspoons powdered gelatin

- ¼ cup raw honey

- 2 tablespoons lemon zest

Cooking Instructions:

1. In a skillet (you can also use a saucepan); heat the water over medium stove flame.

2. Mix in the gelatin and set aside for 10 minutes to thicken.

3. In a bowl (medium size), whisk the milk, lemon juice, honey, and lemon zest.

4. Heat the gelatin mix again and add the milk mixture; stir and heat the mixture.

5. Cool down and refrigerate for about 2 hours until set.

6. Add the mousse into serving bowls.

Nutritional Values (Per Serving):

Calories 318, Fat 11g, Carbohydrates 26g, Fiber 4g, Protein 3g

Quinoa Dessert Bars

Recipe Time: 10 minutes

Serving Size: 8

Diet Type: Gluten Free, Dairy Free, Soy Free, Vegetarian

Ingredients:

- ¼ cup raw honey
- ¼ cup cocoa powder
- ½ cup almond butter
- 4 cups puffed quinoa
- ¼ cup chopped almonds

Cooking Instructions:

1. Grease a square baking dish with some cooking spray.

2. In a skillet (you can also use a saucepan); heat the butter over medium stove flame.

3. Add the honey and cocoa powder. Stir and heat the mix; set aside to cool down.

4. In a mixing bowl, toss the quinoa and almonds.

5. Add the pan mixture. Stir everything together.

6. Add the mixture into the dish and press firmly.

7. Refrigerate for about 1-2 hour. Slice into 16 pieces and serve.

Nutritional Values (Per Serving):

Calories 96, Fat 3g, Carbohydrates 17g, Fiber 1g, Protein 2g

Apple Pear Delight

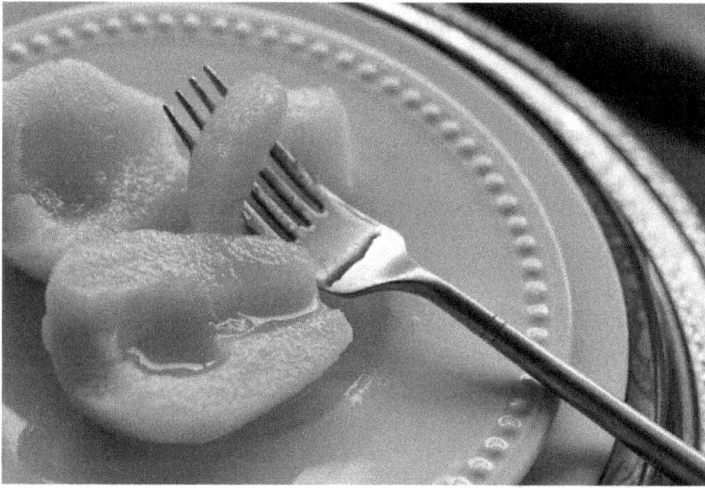

Recipe Time: 25 minutes

Serving Size: 4

Diet Type: Gluten Free, Dairy Free, Soy Free, Nut Free, Vegetarian

Ingredients:

- ¼ cup raw honey

- 1 teaspoon whole cloves

- 4 cups water

- 2 cups unsweetened apple juice

- ½ teaspoon whole cardamom seeds

- 1 teaspoon pure vanilla extract

- 4 pears, peeled, cored and halved

Cooking Instructions:

1. In a skillet (you can also use a saucepan); heat the honey, cloves, water, apple juice, cardamom, and vanilla over medium stove flame.

2. Boil the mix. Reduce the heat to low and simmer for 5 minutes.

3. Add the pear and cover. Simmer for about 8-10 minutes, stirring in between.

4. Add the mixture in serving plates. Serve the pears with the liquid sauce on top.

Nutritional Values (Per Serving):

Calories 238, Fat 0g, Carbohydrates 52g, Fiber 7g, Protein 1g

Pumpkin Pecan Treat

Recipe Time: 10 minutes

Serving Size: 6

Diet Type: Gluten Free, Dairy Free, Soy Free, Nut Free, Vegan, Vegetarian

Ingredients:

1 teaspoon ground cinnamon

½ teaspoon ground ginger

¼ teaspoon ground nutmeg

2 cups canned full-fat coconut milk

1 cup pure pumpkin purée

¼ cup pure maple syrup

Pinch cloves

2 tablespoons chopped pecans, for garnish

Cooking Instructions:

1. In a mixing bowl, whisk the milk, cinnamon, ginger, pumpkin, maple syrup, nutmeg, and cloves.

2. Cover it and refrigerator the bowl for about 2 hours until chilled.

3. Top with the pecans and serve.

Nutritional Values (Per Serving):

Calories 246, Fat 18g, Carbohydrates 17g, Fiber 3g, Protein 4g

Conclusion

Thanks again for taking your valuable time to read this book!

Inflammation fighting foods inspire impactful life changes. They bring true nutrition to your dining table every day. Environmental stimuli affect our gene structure and triggers our body's natural defense through auto-immune response.

Inflammation is the root cause of number of health disorders and ailments. Thankfully, we have the power fight against them by following a wholesome diet. These health diet changes help to relieved the symptoms of auto-immune diseases including arthritis and join pain.

The recipes covered in the book are satiating and full of vibrant flavors. Meal plan is really helpful for beginners as they can consume meals combining various vegetables, spices, meats, and fish varieties.

As you know all the anti-inflammatory foods that you can include in your diet; you can experiment with every day recipes. You can add your choice of ingredients to customize flavors of your preference.

What are you waiting for? Make a trip to your nearby supermarket, stuff your pantry with anti-inflammatory ingredients, and start making these delicious recipes. Thank you and have a great time enjoying these wholesome recipes!

Lastly, if you enjoyed this book, please take the time to review it on Amazon. Your honest feedback would be greatly appreciated. Wish you all the best in achieving vibrancy and optimal health that you all deserve.

Have a great day! Best of luck in all your endeavors.

www.ingramcontent.com/pod-product-compliance
Lightning Source LLC
Chambersburg PA
CBHW051715020426
42333CB00014B/998